FREIDA BAILEY

HOW TO PRACTICE MEDITATION AND YOGA

30 Effective Ways to Practice Meditation and Yoga

Contents

1

INTRODUCTION

The Power of Meditation and Yoga

In the midst of our frenetic lives, when chaos frequently takes center stage, the ancient practices of meditation and yoga shine as beacons of calm, providing a profound medicine for the mind, body, and soul. This essay digs into the enlightening worlds of these age-old disciplines, examining the subtle ways in which they impart the gift of inner harmony, mental clarity, and physical energy.

The Art of Stillness: Meditation as a Path to Inner Peace

Meditation is fundamentally a journey into silence, a mindful halt in the midst of life's tumult. It is more than just a relaxation method; it is a tour into our own psyche. By immersing ourselves in meditation, we tap into a source of peace, where the mind's constant chatter ceases and a profound silence reigns.

Regular meditation has been shown in studies to provide a variety of advantages, including reduced stress and anxiety and improved emotional well-being. The practice promotes mindfulness or awareness that extends to the present moment, developing a strong connection with our thoughts and emotions. Individuals who develop this awareness frequently experience a renewed sense of clarity and resilience in the face of life's obstacles.

The Fluid Poetry of Yoga: A Dance of Body and Spirit.

Yoga complements meditation's quiet by introducing us to the creative dance of the body, a symphony of movement and breath that transcends the physical self's constraints. Beyond the contorted postures is a philosophy that brings together the mind, body, and spirit in a harmonic flow.

Yoga is not a strict fitness plan, but rather a celebration of flexibility, strength, and balance. From the smooth transitions of sun salutations to the grounded quiet of warrior poses, each movement in yoga is a study of the body's capacities and a voyage of self-discovery.

Furthermore, the benefits of yoga go beyond the physical. Regular practice has been associated with better mental health, increased focus, and greater self-awareness. The combination of breath and movement creates a moving meditation, providing a route to awareness that goes well beyond the yoga mat.

A Symbiotic Journey: Integrating Meditation and Yoga.

While meditation and yoga are strong on their own, the ultimate magic happens when they combine to form a symbiotic dance of silence and movement. Meditation serves as an anchor, grounding the mind in serenity, while yoga expresses that inner peace dynamically.

This integration promotes a holistic approach to well-being, with the advantages of mindfulness developed via meditation smoothly woven into the physical postures of yoga. The mind-body link strengthens, and people find themselves not only physically stronger but also mentally resilient, able to face life's obstacles with a newfound serenity.

Beyond Asanas: Navigating the Challenges

Beginning the road of meditation and yoga is not without its challenges. It demands effort, patience, and a willingness to face bodily and mental anguish. However, it is through these obstacles that actual transformation occurs.

Common misconceptions and doubts may occur, but resolving them is an essential part of the process. By acknowledging and conquering these difficulties, practitioners prepare the way for long-term growth and self-discovery.

Cultivating a Lifetime Practice: The Road Ahead

As the journey progresses, it becomes clear that meditation and yoga are not passing trends, but abiding friends for life. Building a supportive group, adjusting practices to one's lifestyle, and growing with the ever-changing landscape of personal growth are all important parts of developing a lifelong practice.

Benefits for Mind and Body

In today's fast-paced world, where stress appears to be an unwelcome companion, the attraction of discovering holistic well-being for both mind and body has led many to the transforming disciplines of meditation and yoga. Beyond the physical postures and moments of quiet, these ancient practices offer a plethora of advantages that reverberate through all areas of our lives.

Calm amid chaos: The mental sanctuary of meditation

One of the significant blessings that meditation bestows on the mind is a haven of peace amid chaos. In a world full of distractions and constant inputs, meditation provides a shelter for the mind to discover stillness. Individuals can cultivate a tranquil mental environment by focusing on their breath and being mindful.

Scientific research has confirmed meditation's beneficial effects on mental health. Regular practitioners report reduced tension, anxiety, and greater emotional well-being. The practice fosters mental resilience, allowing people to tackle challenges with equanimity and emotional equilibrium, even in the face of life's uncertainties.

Physical Vitality with Yoga: Beyond Flexibility and Strength.

While meditation has substantial mental advantages, yoga focuses on the body's physical vigor. It's not just about performing stunning contortions; it's also about improving the body's flexibility, strength, and overall health. The flowing asanas and purposeful breathwork combine to create a dynamic symphony of movement that energizes every muscle and the entire body.

According to research, yoga offers numerous bodily benefits. The tangible effects include improved flexibility and posture, increased muscle strength, and improved respiratory function. Beyond the physical, yoga's careful motions encourage the release of endorphins, which promote a sensation of well-being and vitality.

The Symbiosis of Mind and Body: Integrated Well-Being

The symbiotic interaction between meditation and yoga is what gives them their special power. Meditation acts as an anchor for a peaceful and concentrated mind, while yoga allows you to express your inner calmness through physical movement. Together, they produce a beautiful interplay that goes beyond the confines of simple workout routines or mental activities.

This integration has a significant impact on overall wellness. The mind becomes more aware of the body's signals, and the body becomes a channel for manifesting the tranquility gained via meditation. This holistic approach develops a strong sense of interconnectivity, viewing mental and physical health as inseparable components of a cohesive whole.

Beyond the physical and mental: Spiritual nourishment.

In the pursuit of comprehensive well-being, the benefits extend even to the spiritual components of our existence. Meditation, which is commonly seen as a spiritual activity, offers a path to self-discovery and connection with something higher than oneself. It becomes a trip into the depths of awareness, instilling a sense of purpose and significance in life.

Similarly, yoga, which has its roots in ancient spiritual traditions, encourages people to explore the spiritual aspects of their lives. The meditative movements and breathwork create a sacred environment for reflection, allowing practitioners to connect with themselves and the larger cosmos.

Cultivating a Lifelong Sense of Wellbeing

As people begin to incorporate meditation and yoga into their lives, the advantages emerge as long-lasting attributes that build a lifelong feeling of well-being. The tranquil mind, vital body, and nourished soul become companions on the path of self-discovery, guiding people through life's complications with resilience, grace, and an unwavering sense of harmony.

2

Chapter One: Getting Started

Setting the Right Mindset

In the complicated fabric of life, the lens through which we see the world frequently determines the course of our trip. Mindset, the mental framework that determines our beliefs and actions, has an unprecedented impact on personal development, resilience, and general well-being. In this exploration, we will delve into the profound world of developing the correct attitude, understanding its relevance, and revealing ways for cultivating a mental landscape favorable to personal transformation.

Understanding the Power of Mindset.

The concept of mentality, popularised by psychologist Carol S. Dweck, is more than just a psychological construct; it serves as a compass for our responses to difficulties, failures, and accomplishments. At its foundation, mindset reflects the beliefs we have about ourselves and our skills, which influence the direction of our lives in subtle but powerful ways.

A. Fixed vs. Growth Mindset: The Foundation of Perspective.

The debate revolves around the distinction between a fixed and a developing mindset. A fixed mindset regards abilities as innate traits, causing people to avoid difficulties and interpret failure as a reflection of their essential capabilities. A growth mindset, on the other hand, sees problems as learning opportunities and believes that skills can be acquired through hard work and dedication.

Understanding this fundamental distinction is critical because it lays the framework for understanding the influence attitude has on personal development. Individuals who cultivate a growth mindset gain resilience, adaptability, and the ability to continuously develop themselves.

The Impact of Mindset on Personal Growth

A. Accepting Challenges as Opportunities

A growth mentality views setbacks as stepping stones rather than insurmountable obstacles. Challenges serve as accelerators for progress, encouraging people to stretch their talents, learn from setbacks, and ultimately emerge stronger. This shift in perspective encourages a proactive approach to life, in which challenges are welcomed as chances for self-discovery and progress.

B. Managing Failures with Resilience

In the growth mindset paradigm, failure is viewed as a temporary setback on the way to mastery rather than a verdict on one's ability. Individuals with a growth mentality recover from failures with tenacity, seeing them as helpful input rather than defining moments. This resilience becomes a pillar of personal development, enabling people to overcome hardship and emerge wiser and more resilient.

C. Fostering a Love of Learning.

A growth mindset fosters a passion for learning that extends beyond formal education. It is a mindset that sees every event as a chance to acquire new abilities, widen perspectives, and progress as a person. This passion for learning creates a self-reinforcing cycle, moving people towards ongoing development and dynamic engagement with their surroundings.

Strategies for cultivating a growth mindset.

A. Self-Awareness: The First Step to Transformation

Self-awareness is the foundation for creating a growth mentality. It requires a thorough grasp of one's beliefs, mental habits, and reactions. Individuals might begin their change journey by studying their inner dialogue and identifying stuck mentality patterns.

B. Taking on Challenges Deliberately

Deliberately seeking out obstacles is a proactive method for developing a growth mindset. Individuals who willingly move beyond their comfort zones expose themselves to new situations that need adaptation and growth. This deliberate response to challenges rewires the brain, reinforcing the notion that effort leads to progress.

C. Changing Views on Effort and Criticism.

In the sphere of a growth mentality, effort serves as a currency of growth. It is critical to shift the mindset from viewing effort as a sign of weakness to one of mastery. Similarly, accepting constructive criticism as feedback for progress rather than a personal assault helps to turn setbacks into chances for growth.

D. Celebrating Progress, not Just Achievements.

Celebrating progress is a game changer in a culture that is frequently focused on the end product. Recognizing and appreciating incremental progress, no matter how minor fosters the notion that the journey is as important as the destination. This mindset adjustment supports a long-term commitment to growth.

Mindset in Action: Real-World Examples

A. Success Stories for Growth Mindset Pioneers

Real-life examples demonstrate how a development mindset can improve lives. From Thomas Edison's dedication in creating the light bulb to J.K. Rowling's bravery in overcoming rejection, these anecdotes demonstrate that failures are not obstacles, but detours on the path to success.

B. Cultural Paradigms and Mindset Changes

Examining cultural paradigms also provides information about the impact of attitude. Cultures that respect hard work, perseverance, and learning are more likely to promote a collective growth attitude. Individuals who grasp the cultural impacts on attitude can negotiate society's expectations while remaining true to their unique development journey.

Challenges of Developing a Growth Mindset

A. Overcoming Fixed Mindset Habits.

Breaking free from ingrained fixed mentality behaviors necessitates conscious effort. Procrastination, avoidance of challenges, and self-limiting attitudes are prevalent hurdles. Recognizing and changing unhealthy habits with growth-oriented behaviors is an ongoing process that requires self-reflection and commitment.

B. Addressing External Influences

External forces, such as societal expectations and negative feedback, might make it difficult to sustain a growth mentality. Building resilience to external challenges entails cultivating a strong sense of self, adhering to personal principles, and finding support from a community that encourages growth and learning.

Creating a Sacred Space for Practice

The concept of a sacred space is extremely important in our fast-paced daily life. It extends beyond the physical environment, becoming a haven for reflection, self-discovery, and mindful practice.

The essence of a sacred space.

A. Beyond the Physical: Nurturing Spirituality

Creating a sacred space is more than just design or aesthetics; it is a conscious act of cultivating the spiritual aspects of our existence. It is an intentional decision to create a haven where external noise diminishes and interior harmony flourishes. Whether you're practicing meditation, yoga, or another sort of introspective practice, the environment you inhabit catalyzes connecting with yourself and the divine.

B. Intentionality in Design: Aligning the External and Internal

The architecture of a sacred area reflects intentionality. Every element, from colors and textures to lighting and décor, adds to the ambiance. The goal is to match the exterior environment with the internal state, resulting in a seamless flow of the physical and intangible. This deliberate design promotes the transition from the outside world to the inner sphere of concentrated practice.

Choosing the Right Space.

A. Designing Spaces to Meet Individual Needs

The perfect sacred space is a deeply personal decision. It could be a separate room, a corner in a common space, or an outdoor nook. The objective is to design the environment around individual needs and tastes. Whether it's a minimalist setting with natural components or a cozy hideaway studded with important artifacts, the chosen place should strike a chord with the practitioner, generating feelings of tranquility and connection.

B. Practical considerations: accessibility and comfort.

Practical concerns play a role in determining the best space. Accessibility, comfort, and proximity to nature all contribute to a sacred space's effectiveness. It should be a welcoming environment in which practitioners can smoothly integrate their practice into their daily activities.

Elements of a Sacred Space

A. Lighting: Illuminating the Inward Journey

Lighting has a tremendous influence on the aura of a sacred area. Soft, diffused lighting produces a soothing ambiance by reducing stark contrasts and encouraging a sense of calm. When natural light is present, it serves as a conduit for a more in-depth connection with the surroundings.

B. Colours and Textures: Harmony of the Senses

The color and texture scheme determines the emotional tone of the room. Earthy tones frequently produce a sense of grounding, but calming blues and greens create a peaceful atmosphere. Textures, whether in the shape of cushions, rugs, or natural materials, add to the multimodal experience and help practitioners stay in the present moment.

C. Symbols and Artefacts: Evoking Meaningful Presence

Symbols and artifacts can convey a deeper sense of meaning. These pieces, whether they are loved mementos, spiritual icons, or symbols that correspond to particular beliefs, add intention and value to the area. They serve as reminders of the practice's objective, keeping practitioners focused and mindful.

D. Plants and Nature: Integrating Organic

Bringing nature into the sacred place fosters a connection with the organic world. Indoor plants not only improve air quality, but they also represent growth, rejuvenation, and the cycle of life. Nature-inspired noises, like running water or rustling leaves, can help to enhance the immersive experience.

Rituals & Ceremonies: Strengthening the Connection

A. Setting the Tone Through Rituals

Incorporating rituals into holy space practice creates a conducive environment for focused reflection. This could entail lighting candles, burning incense, or taking a period of quiet thought. Rituals serve as transitions, indicating to the mind that it is time to move from the outside world to the inner sanctuary.

B. Personalising Practices with Ceremonies

Ceremonies in sacred spaces give a sense of personalization to the activity. Whether it's a daily affirmation, a gratitude ritual, or a symbolic gesture, these ceremonies strengthen the connection to the space and give the practice a sense of purpose.

Creating a Mobile Sacred Space: Adjusting to Change

A. The Idea of a Portable Sanctuary

Recognizing the changing nature of life, the concept of a movable sacred space becomes useful. A mobile altar, meditation cushion, or symbolic item can function as a portable sanctuary, allowing practitioners to take the essence of their sacred space with them wherever they go. This adaptability guarantees that the benefits of mindful practice are accessible regardless of external circumstances.

B. Mindful Practices Beyond the Designated Space.

Extending mindful activities beyond the specified sacred site strengthens the idea that the sanctuary dwells within, rather than in a specific physical location. Integrating mindfulness into daily activities, from attentive walking to aware breathing, bridges the gap between the sacred place and the greater canvas of life.

Overcoming Challenges in Creating a Sacred Space

A. Space constraints and adaptability.

Not everyone has the luxury of a private room or a large space. Adapting to space limits requires imagination and a willingness to make the best of what is available. With careful planning, small niches, outdoor places, or even a reserved chair can be transformed into powerful sacred spaces.

B. Distractions & External Influences

External influences and distractions make it difficult to maintain the space's sacredness. Establishing boundaries, expressing the importance of the area to others, and including soundproofing measures can all contribute to a favorable environment for concentrated practice.

The Transformational Impact of Sacred Spaces

A. Improved focus and presence.

A well-designed sacred place serves as a focal point, directing attention and intent. It serves as a haven from distractions, allowing practitioners to fully immerse themselves in the present moment. The increased attention and presence developed in the sacred place extends beyond the practice, influencing daily activities with conscious awareness.

B. Stress Reduction and Emotional Wellness

The purposeful design of a sacred space promotes stress reduction and emotional well-being. The relaxing components, ranging from lighting to symbolic artifacts, create an environment that relaxes the nervous system and promotes emotional resilience. Regular practice in this place becomes a self-care ritual, a little break from the responsibilities of the outside world.

C. Deepening the Spiritual Connection

For people on a spiritual path, a holy space serves as a conduit for a deeper connection with the divine or higher self. It becomes a sacred portal through which people can explore their inner landscapes, seek guidance, and feel a sense of connection with the sublime.

Essential Tools and Accessories

Meditation and yoga are ageless techniques that help people towards comprehensive well-being and inner tranquility. As you go on these transforming trips, it is critical to choose the correct tools and accessories. This article goes into the important tools and accessories for meditation and yoga, examining the impact they can have on your practice and overall experience.

Meditation: Tools for Stillness and Presence.

A. Meditation Cushion or Pillow: Enhancing Comfort and Posture.

The modest meditation cushion or pillow is important to a relaxing meditation practice. This seemingly simple addition is essential for improving comfort while sitting for lengthy periods. It promotes appropriate posture by letting the spine to naturally align and elevating the hips, which reduces strain on the lower back. Whether in a designated meditation area or a spare corner of your home, selecting a cushion that meets your comfort needs ensures a more immersed and concentrated meditation experience.

B. Meditation Bench Provides Flexibility and Support.

A meditation seat offers a varied option to sitting flat on the floor. These seats encourage a kneeling position, reducing pressure on the knees and ankles. Their portability enables practitioners to create a meditation area in a variety of venues, offering flexibility to the practice.

C. Meditation Timer or App: Guided Mindful Sessions

In the digital era, meditation timers or apps are essential aids for keeping organization and attention during sessions. Whether you like the classic sound of a singing bowl or the instruction of a soothing voice, these instruments can help you build a rhythm in your practice. Set intervals or select from a variety of meditation themes to enrich your sessions and promote mindfulness.

Yoga Tools for Flow and Alignment.

A. Yoga Mat: The Foundation for Grounded Practice.

The yoga mat serves as the foundation of your practice, offering a non-slip surface and cushioning for joints when in poses. The correct mat provides stability in balancing positions and increases comfort during floor activities. With so many variations available, from eco-friendly materials to extra-thick designs, choosing a mat that suits your needs provides a stable and joyful yoga experience.

B. Yoga Blocks: Enhancing Strength and Flexibility

Yoga blocks are adaptable props that give support and stability to poses. These blocks are suitable for practitioners of all skill levels, whether used to bring the floor closer in standing poses or to aid in obtaining perfect alignment. Because of their lightweight and portable character, they are excellent instruments for developing personalized and adaptive yoga practices.

C. Yoga Strap for Deeper Stretches and Increased Flexibility

A yoga strap can help practitioners deepen stretches and improve flexibility.

These basic yet efficient aids help achieve perfect alignment, particularly in positions that require reaching or binding. Incorporating a yoga strap into your practice allows for progressive advancement, which promotes ease and attention.

D. Bolster encourages relaxation and restorative practices.

For restorative yoga or periods of relaxation, a bolster is an essential item. When placed under the knees, lower back, or neck, it gives mild support while encouraging relaxation and comfort. Bolsters are especially useful for restorative poses and meditation sessions, as they create a caring atmosphere in which the body and mind may relax.

Common Tools for Both Practices

A. Essential Oils and Diffusers: Enhancing the Atmosphere

Making a pleasant and peaceful environment is essential for both meditation and yoga practices. Essential oils and diffusers add to the mood by infusing the environment with relaxing scents. Scents such as lavender, eucalyptus, and sandalwood can help you relax, focus, and be aware. Selecting scents that speak to you gives a sensory depth to your practice, encouraging a greater connection with the present moment.

B. Comfortable Attire: Promotes Freedom of Movement

While not a physical instrument, wearing comfortable and breathable clothing is essential for free mobility during yoga and meditation. The appropriate clothes allow you to concentrate on your practice without distractions, fostering a sensation of freedom and relaxation. To improve your overall experience, prioritize comfort while choosing loose-fitting yoga trousers, a breathable top, or specialized meditation clothes.

C. Water Bottle: Staying hydrated and mindful.

Both meditation and yoga benefit greatly from adequate hydration. Having a separate water bottle nearby acts as a practical reminder to stay hydrated throughout your practice. Choosing a reusable bottle coincides with eco-friendly ideas, resulting in a comprehensive approach to well-being that goes beyond individual practice.

Mindful Selection: Personalising Your Practice

A. Listening to Your Body and Preferences.

Each person's experience with meditation and yoga is unique. Listening to your body and understanding your preferences are essential for making informed tool and accessory choices. Experimenting with numerous alternatives helps you to personalize your practice to your comfort level, goals, and personal preferences.

B. Considering Your Practice Environment

The atmosphere in which you practice has a huge impact on your whole experience. When selecting equipment and accessories, take into account the available area, lighting, and ambiance. Whether you're constructing a specialised meditation nook or a multipurpose yoga studio, aligning your equipment with your practice space improves the harmony between the physical and mental parts of your practice.

3

Chapter Two :The Art of Meditation

Mindfulness Techniques

In today's fast-paced world, mindfulness emerges as a guiding light, providing a sanctuary of presence amidst the chaos. This article delves into the various mindfulness techniques that cultivate awareness, improve well-being, and foster a profound connection with the present moment.

Understanding Mindfulness: A Foundation for Well-Being.

A. Essence of Mindfulness: Embracing the Now

At its essence, mindfulness is a state of heightened awareness, an intentional decision to focus one's attention on the present moment without judgment. Mindfulness, which has its roots in ancient contemplative traditions, has crossed cultural barriers to become a transforming practice that is widely adopted around the world. It entails developing an open, receptive attitude towards one's experiences, be they thoughts, emotions, or feelings.

B. Mindfulness vs. Mindlessness: Understanding the Differences

Mindlessness, the default state of autopilot living, frequently isolates people from the richness of their experiences. Mindfulness, on the other hand, is a conscious choice to actively participate in the unfolding of each moment. It is a shift from habitual response patterns, encouraging people to conduct their lives with greater clarity and intentionality.

Mindfulness Techniques for Daily Living

A. Mindful Breathing: An Anchor for the Present

One of the most important mindfulness exercises is conscious breathing. The breath serves as a constant connection to the current moment. Mindful breathing entails paying attention to the sensations of each breath: the rise and fall of the chest, and the sensation of air passing through the nose. This approach not only relaxes the mind but also connects you directly to the ever-changing flow of the moment.

B. Body Scan Meditation: A Journey to Awareness

Body scan meditation encourages practitioners to investigate the sensations in each region of their bodies systematically. Individuals gain a better understanding of bodily feelings, stress, and areas of comfort by focusing their attention on different body locations. This approach encourages a mind-body connection, which improves relaxation and anchoring in the present.

C. Loving-Kindness Meditation: Developing Compassion

Loving-kindness Meditation, also known as Metta meditation, is a practice that focuses on developing feelings of love and compassion. Practitioners express well wishes to themselves, loved ones, acquaintances, and even people with whom they may disagree. This strategy not only promotes kindness but also increases empathy and connection.

D. Mindful Walking: Integrating Movement with Awareness

Mindful walking entails focusing conscious attention on the act of walking.

Each stride provides an opportunity for awareness, with a focus on the sensations of lifting, moving, and placing the feet. Mindful walking may be practiced in a variety of circumstances, making it a dynamic approach to incorporate mindfulness into everyday life while engaging with the world in a thoughtful and grounded manner.

E. Mindful Eating: Enjoying the Experience

Mindful eating transforms the act of eating into a sensory experience. Individuals develop a stronger bond with their food by paying attention to its taste, texture, and scent. Mindful eating also improves an awareness of hunger and fullness cues, establishing a healthy relationship with food.

Mindfulness-Based Stress Reduction (MBSR): A Comprehensive Approach.

A: The Origins and Principles of MBSR

Dr. Jon Kabat-Zinn developed Mindfulness-Based Stress Reduction (MBSR), a structured program that combines various mindfulness techniques to create a holistic approach to stress reduction and overall well-being. MBSR, which is based on Buddhist meditation practices, has garnered international acclaim for its ability to reduce stress and anxiety while also increasing resilience.

B. Bringing Mindfulness into Daily Life

The MBSR program consists of guided mindfulness meditations, body scan activities, and yoga practices. Participants eventually learn to incorporate mindfulness into their daily lives, using the strategies to deal with stressors and obstacles. Individuals who practice mindfulness daily arm themselves with significant tools for dealing with life's complexity in a calm and focused manner.

Mindfulness in Clinical Settings: Mindfulness-Based Cognitive Therapy (MBCT).

A. Managing Recurrent Depression and Anxiety.

Mindfulness-Based Cognitive Therapy (MBCT) is an empirically supported treatment method that aims to prevent depressive episodes from recurring. MBCT, which combines aspects of cognitive therapy with mindfulness techniques, teaches patients how to interrupt the loop of negative thought patterns that contribute to depression and anxiety.

B. The Integration of Mindfulness and Cognitive Therapy

MBCT emphasizes the practice of mindfulness to become aware of automatic thought patterns that can lead to depression recurrence. Individuals gain agency in reacting to situations when they develop a nonjudgmental awareness of their ideas and feelings. This integrated method allows people to notice their cognitive processes without being enmeshed in them, which promotes a better sense of well-being.

Technology and mindfulness: Apps and guided meditations

A. The Rise of Mindfulness Apps.

The digital era has seen the rise of mindfulness apps, which put guided meditations and mindfulness exercises at users' fingertips. Apps such as Headspace, Calm, and Insight Timer offer accessible venues for individuals to engage in their mindfulness journey. These tools include guided sessions, meditation timers, and progress tracking, making mindfulness more accessible in our technologically driven world.

B. Guided Meditations: A Companion to Practitioners

Guided meditations, whether delivered through apps, online platforms, or in-person meetings, provide a structured approach for people new to mindfulness or looking for diversity in their practice. Experienced meditation instructors guide practitioners through focused exercises, assisting them in developing the skills required to cultivate mindfulness on their own.

Challenges of Mindfulness Practice

A. Patience and Persistence: Managing Initial Discomfort

Cultivating mindfulness is not without challenges. Many people feel uncomfortable or restless at first when attempting to quiet their minds. Patience and tenacity are essential as practitioners overcome these initial challenges, acknowledging that the practice is an ongoing journey of self-discovery.

B. Balancing Technology with Mindfulness Practices

While mindfulness applications and digital tools provide useful information, it is critical to strike a balance between technology use and direct, unmediated experiences. The idea is to integrate mindfulness into daily living rather than relying primarily on external reminders. Mindfulness is not passive consumption; rather, it is an active participation in the present moment.

Mindfulness in Everyday Life: Beyond Formal Practices

A. Informal Mindfulness: Turning Awareness into Action

Beyond formal activities, mindfulness permeates the fabric of daily life through informal practices. This entails bringing conscious awareness to everyday activities such as washing dishes and walking the dog. Informal mindfulness supports the idea that mindfulness is a way of being in the world, rather than a certain time or place.

B. Mindful Communication: Nurturing Connection.

Mindfulness extends into interpersonal interactions via mindful communication. This includes remaining fully present and attentive throughout talks, developing empathy, and responding thoughtfully rather than reactively. Mindful speaking promotes deeper connections while reducing the possibility of misunderstandings.

The Transformative Impact of Mindfulness Practices

A. Mental and Emotional Wellbeing

M.indfulness has frequently been shown in scientific studies to improve mental and emotional well-being. Regular mindfulness practice has been linked to lower levels of stress, anxiety, and depression-related symptoms. The development of mindfulness skills enables people to face problems with more resilience and emotional balance.

B. Enhanced Cognitive Functioning

Mindfulness activities have demonstrated positive impacts on cognitive performance. According to research, mindfulness can increase attention, memory, and decision-making skills. Regular mindfulness meditation improves focus and cognitive flexibility.

C. Physical Health Benefits

The mind-body link inherent in mindfulness techniques promotes physical wellness. Mindfulness has been associated with reduced blood pressure, better sleep quality, and improved immune system performance. Reducing stress-related physiological responses contributes to improved overall physical well-being.

Mindfulness in the Workplace: Developing a Resilient Culture

A: Stress Reduction and Employee Well-Being

Recognizing the importance of mindfulness for individual well-being, many organizations are implementing mindfulness programs in the workplace.

These programs aim to reduce workplace stress, boost employee resilience, and build a healthier business culture. Mindfulness training can help to boost job satisfaction and foster a more positive work atmosphere.

B. Increasing Focus and Productivity

Mindfulness in the workplace is linked to increased focus and productivity. Organizations can foster a culture of sustained attention and innovative problem-solving by encouraging employees to take thoughtful breaks and implementing brief mindfulness activities into their workdays.

Breathing Exercises

In the symphony of body functions, breathing takes center stage as a vital rhythm. Beyond its physiological requirement, breathing has significant ramifications for our mental, emotional, and physical health. This article delves deeply into breathing exercises, examining the various strategies that unlock the transforming power of conscious breathing.

The Basic Essence of Breathing: More Than Just Survival

A. Unconscious Breathing: A Vital Constant

Breathing is an autonomic process that runs smoothly in the background of our daily lives. In its most basic form, breathing provides life support by allowing the exchange of oxygen and carbon dioxide. The respiratory system functions on autopilot, reacting to the body's needs without conscious effort.

B. Beyond Survival: The Mind-Body Connection.

However, the importance of breathing goes beyond survival. Conscious and intentional breathing serves as a link between the conscious and unconscious parts of our being. It is an effective method for reducing stress, cultivating mindfulness, and developing a stronger connection with the present moment.

The Science of Breath: How Conscious Breathing Influences the Body.

A. Diaphragmatic and Thoracic Breathing: Respiratory Mechanics

Understanding the mechanics of respiration is critical for recognizing the effectiveness of breathing exercises. The diaphragm, a dome-shaped muscle beneath the lungs, is crucial to breathing. During inhalation, the diaphragm contracts, forming a vacuum that sucks air into the lungs. Exhalation happens when the diaphragm relaxes and expels air from the lungs.

Thoracic breathing, which is characterized by shallow breaths primarily involving the chest, is a common pattern seen in stressed or nervous conditions. In contrast, diaphragmatic breathing, also known as abdominal or deep breathing, fully activates the diaphragm, resulting in a slower and more rhythmic breath.

B. The Autonomic Nervous System: Integrating Breath and Emotion

The autonomic nerve system (ANS), which includes the sympathetic and parasympathetic branches, is critical for controlling physiological responses to stress. Conscious breathing serves as a link between the autonomic nervous system and emotional health. Deep diaphragmatic breathing activates the parasympathetic nervous system, which induces a relaxation response while counteracting the sympathetic nervous system's stress reaction.

Breathing Exercises: Tapestry of Techniques

A. Diaphragmatic Breathing is the foundation of calm.

Diaphragmatic breathing is the cornerstone for many breathing exercises. To practice diaphragmatic breathing, sit or lie down in a comfortable position. Place one hand on your chest, and the other on your abdomen. Inhale deeply through your nose, feeling your abdomen rise as your diaphragm contracts. Exhale slowly through your lips, feeling your stomach drop. This technique develops calm and centeredness by engaging the diaphragm and slowing the breath.

B. Box Breathing: Promoting Balance

Box breathing, also known as square breathing, is a technique that focuses on equal durations for inhalation, holding the breath, expiration, and another breath-holding phase. Begin by breathing for four counts, holding your breath for four counts, exhaling for four counts, and repeating for four counts. This rhythmic pattern helps to balance the neural system, promoting a sense of equilibrium and attention.

C. 4-7-8 Breathing: Relaxing Breath

Dr. Andrew Weil developed the 4-7-8 breathing technique, which consists of inhaling through the nose for four counts, holding the breath for seven counts, and expelling through the mouth for eight counts. This exercise is intended to promote relaxation by extending the exhalation phase, resulting in a release of tension and a calming influence on the nervous system.

D. Alternate Nostril Breathing (Nadi Shodhana): Balancing Energy

Alternate nostril breathing, which originated in yogic traditions, is a practice that seeks to balance the flow of energy throughout the body. Sit comfortably, with your spine straight. Close your right nostril with your thumb and take a deep breath through your left. Close the left nostril with your right ring finger and exhale through the right nostril. Inhale via the right nostril, close it, then exhale through the left. This pattern continues with alternating nostrils. Nadi Shodhana is thought to improve mental clarity and balance the two hemispheres of the brain.

E. Resonant Breathing (Coherent Breathing): Coordinating with Heart Rate Variability.

Resonant or coherent breathing entails keeping a steady breathing rate that corresponds to heart rate variability. The ideal rate is usually between five and six breaths per minute. The synchronization of breath and heart rate variability improves autonomic nervous system coherence, which fosters emotional balance and resilience.

Mind-Body Harmony: The Psychological Effects of Breathing Exercises

A: Stress Reduction and Anxiety Management

One of the main advantages of mindful breathing exercises is their capacity to reduce the effects of stress and anxiety. Deep diaphragmatic breathing activates the parasympathetic nerve system, which counteracts the physiological stress response, resulting in lowered cortisol levels and a sense of calm.

B. Improved focus and concentration.

Conscious breathing has a direct effect on cognitive functioning. Breathing exercises improve attention and concentration by relaxing and clearing the mind. Certain techniques, such as box breathing, have a rhythmic aspect that coincides with cognitive processes and promotes mental clarity.

C. Emotional Regulation and Mood Enhancement

The relationship between breath and emotion is profound. Breathing exercises are a useful tool for emotional regulation, allowing people to navigate and respond to emotions with more awareness and calm. Conscious breathing has a relaxing impact that improves mood and emotional well-being.

Breathing Exercises for Specialised Practices

A. Pranayama: Harnessing Life Force

In yogic traditions, pranayama is the practice of controlling one's breath. It includes a variety of breathing exercises aimed to control the flow of prana, or life force, throughout the body. Ujjayi breath, Kapalabhati breath, and Bhramari breath are examples of pranayama practices, each of which has a specific goal such as energizing the body, purifying the respiratory system, and producing meditative states.

B. Holotropic Breathwork: Exploring Altered States.

Dr. Stanislav Grof invented Holotropic Breathwork, a therapeutic practice that uses intensive and rhythmic breathing to induce altered states of consciousness. Participants practice deep, continuous breathing to reach the unconscious mind and enable emotional discharge. Holotropic Breathwork is frequently practiced in a facilitated group environment.

The Role of Breath in Meditation: A Gateway to Presence.

A. Breath Awareness Meditation: Anchoring in the Present

Breath awareness. Meditation, a fundamental practice in many contemplative traditions, is focusing attention on the breath. Whether watching the natural flow of breath or counting inhalations and exhalations, this practice promotes mindfulness by focusing attention on the present moment. The breath becomes a portal to increased awareness and a calm mind.

B. Integrating Breath and Mindfulness Practices

Breathing exercises are smoothly integrated with mindfulness techniques, emphasizing the relationship between breath and present-moment awareness. Mindful breathing promotes a nonjudgmental awareness of ideas, sensations, and emotions that arise during the exercise. This integration promotes deeper mindfulness, allowing people to create a more profound sense of presence.

Addressing Common Challenges in Breathing Exercises

A. Overcome Shallow Breathing Habits

Many people acquire shallow breathing patterns, particularly in response to stress or lengthy durations of sitting. Overcoming these behaviors requires conscious effort and consistent practice of deep diaphragmatic breathing. Using techniques such as diaphragmatic breathing and box breathing can help the body retrain itself to breathe more naturally and efficiently.

B. Patience and Consistency are the keys to long-term benefits.

Breathing exercises provide transformative advantages over time with persistent practice. Patience is essential as people traverse the learning curve and create a routine. Incorporating breathing exercises into daily life, whether as part of a morning ritual, during stressful situations, or before bedtime, increases their effectiveness over time.

Breathing Exercises For Specific Populations

A. Athletes' Performance Enhancement

Breathing exercises are vital for sports performance. Techniques such as rhythmic breathing synchronize with physical activity, improving oxygen intake and energy efficiency. Athletes frequently include breathwork into their training regimens to improve endurance, attention, and recovery.

B. Children and Stress Reduction.

Breathing exercises are an effective strategy for children to handle stress and develop emotional resilience. Simple techniques, such as balloon breathing, in which youngsters imagine inflating and deflating a balloon with their breath, make breathwork more accessible and pleasurable. These approaches help children navigate their emotions and develop coping skills.

Overcoming Common Challenges

In the rich tapestry of life, problems appear as unavoidable threads woven flawlessly into the fabric of our journey. From the struggles of personal development to the intricacies of daily life, managing common challenges necessitates a sophisticated strategy based on resilience, self-awareness, and adaptive techniques.

Understanding the nature of challenges: inherent and transformative.

A. Growth-Promoting Challenges

Challenges, in their various forms, can act as catalysts for personal and social development. They encourage introspection, self-discovery, and the development of resilience. While initially intimidating, overcoming obstacles can lead to transformative experiences that shape people into more resilient, compassionate, and capable creatures.

B: The Unpredictability of Life's Journey

Life's journey is naturally unpredictable, with seasons of joy, adversity, and all in between. Challenges originate from both external and internal fights, resulting in a dynamic environment in which adaptation becomes a key asset. Recognizing the inevitability of obstacles encourages people to approach them with curiosity and a desire to learn.

Common Challenges in the Human Experience:

A. Emotional Turbulence: Navigating the Depths of Feelings

Emotional problems are an inherent aspect of the human experience. From the highs of joy and love to the lows of grief and terror, emotions weave a complex tapestry of human existence. Managing emotional turmoil entails developing emotional intelligence, accepting feelings without judgment, and creating appropriate coping methods. Accepting emotions as vital communicators helps increase self-awareness and emotional resilience.

B. Relationship Dynamics: Creating Bridges Between Differences

Interpersonal problems are woven into the fabric of all relationships, whether family, romantic, or professional. Communication failures, disagreements, and misaligned expectations are common roadblocks. Building bridges between these issues necessitates active listening, empathy, and a willingness to grasp different points of view. Healthy partnerships require open communication, clear limits, and mutual respect.

C. Self-Doubt and the Inner Critic: Developing Self-Compassion

The inner landscape frequently contains the problems of self-doubt and the unwavering inner critic. Overcoming these difficulties entails developing self-compassion, questioning negative self-talk, and acknowledging one's inherent value. Embracing vulnerability and admitting flaws are critical elements in establishing a foundation of self-esteem and resilience against the internal difficulties that can stymie personal growth.

D. Career and Ambition: Managing Professional Challenges

Professional problems, such as job transitions, workplace dynamics, or achieving lofty goals, are inherent in the road of personal and professional development. Career problems can be overcome via continual learning, adaptation, networking, and persistence in the face of failures. Maintaining a growth mindset encourages taking a proactive response to work problems, changing them into opportunities for skill development and career advancement.

E. Health and Well-Being: Continuing a Holistic Approach

Health issues, whether physical or emotional, are intrinsic to the human experience. Navigating health challenges requires a comprehensive approach that considers physical, mental, and emotional well-being. Seeking expert help, adopting good lifestyle practices, and cultivating a positive attitude all contribute to resilience in the face of health issues.

Strategies for Overcoming Common Challenges.

A. Developing Resilience: The Art of Bouncing Back

Resilience is the ability to recover from adversity and can be developed via intentional activities. Building resilience entails cultivating a good attitude, viewing setbacks as chances for progress, and keeping a sense of purpose. Accepting setbacks as part of the journey promotes adaptation and increases the ability to negotiate life's twists and turns.

B. Developing Emotional Intelligence as a Relationship Compass

Emotional intelligence, the ability to recognize and manage one's own emotions and empathize with others, is a cornerstone for overcoming interpersonal issues. Self-reflection, active listening, and empathy are all necessary for developing emotional intelligence. Individuals who understand and regulate their emotions can promote healthier relationships and negotiate conflicts more effectively.

C. Mindfulness and present-moment awareness: anchoring in the now

Mindfulness, or the practice of being fully present in the present moment, is an effective strategy for overcoming problems. Individuals can break free from past regrets and future fears by focusing on the current moment. Mindfulness techniques, such as meditation and conscious breathing, promote self-awareness, reduce stress, and create a basis for confronting issues with a clear and focused mind.

D. Goal Setting and Adaptability: Managing Professional Challenges

In the arena of professional problems, goal setting and adaptation are crucial. Clearly defined goals give a road map, whereas adaptability provides for flexibility in the face of unexpected challenges. Balancing ambition with a realistic evaluation of resources and schedules allows people to approach job obstacles intelligently. Adopting a growth mindset encourages constant learning, allowing individuals to adapt in tandem with the ever-changing nature of their professional terrain.

E. Seeking Support and Connection: The Strength of Unity

It might be intimidating to face challenges alone. Seeking help from friends, family, or professionals builds a network of connections that gives both emotional and practical support. Whether dealing with personal, professional, or health issues, the strength found in unity and shared experiences may be a tremendous motivator and source of resilience.

Importance of Self-Reflection as a Compass for Growth

A. The Mirror of Self-Reflection: Revealing Inner Truths

Self-reflection is an effective strategy for personal development, allowing people to uncover underlying truths and acquire clarity about their beliefs, aspirations, and motives. Regular self-reflection includes introspection, journaling, and mindfulness. It acts as a compass, leading people through the complexities of issues by increasing self-awareness and facilitating deliberate decision-making.

B. Learning from Setbacks: Turning Challenges Into Wisdom

Setbacks are an unavoidable aspect of overcoming obstacles. Instead of perceiving setbacks as failures, seeing them as chances for learning and progress changes the narrative. Learning from setbacks entails analyzing past events, recognizing lessons, and applying discovered knowledge to future endeavors. Each failure serves as a learning experience that leads to resilience and mastery.

Cultivating a Positive Mindset: Growing the Seeds of Optimism

A positive outlook is an effective ally in conquering obstacles. Cultivating optimism entails reframing negative ideas, concentrating on solutions rather than problems, and recognizing progress, no matter how tiny. Individuals who cultivate a positive outlook develop a mental framework that allows them to meet problems with perseverance, creativity, and confidence in their capacity to overcome adversity.

4

Chapter Three: Yoga Demystified

Basics for Beginners

Embarking on a new adventure, whether it's to learn a new skill, pursue a hobby, or explore a new field of knowledge, is an exciting but sometimes daunting experience. As newcomers approach the threshold of possibility, comprehending the fundamentals serves as a compass to guide their first steps.

The Beginner's Mind: A Foundation for Growth.

A. Promoting Curiosity and Openness.

The essence of the "beginner's mind" – a Zen Buddhist idea – is at the heart of every good beginning. Cultivating a beginner's mindset entails approaching each encounter with curiosity and openness, free of preconceived notions or judgments. Embracing the unfamiliar with a fresh viewpoint enables newcomers to absorb new information, skills, and perspectives without the burden of assumptions.

B. Accepting the Learning Curve

Beginners must understand that a learning curve is an important aspect of any new endeavour. The early phases may be difficult, and progress may appear slow, but understanding that it is all part of the process promotes resilience. When challenges emerge, recognizing them as opportunities for growth rather than impediments fosters a positive and empowered perspective.

Setting Clear Intentions: Define Goals and Expectations.

A. Clarifying Personal Goals

Before embarking on a new endeavour, it is important to establish clear goals. What exactly does success look like? What talents or expertise do you want to acquire? Setting personal goals gives newcomers direction and purpose, allowing them to adapt their learning experience to match their aspirations.

B. Managing Expectations.

While enthusiasm is necessary, regulating expectations is equally important. Recognizing that development may be slow, setbacks may occur, and competence takes time to acquire avoids unnecessary frustration. Realistic expectations lay the groundwork for a patient and sustained approach to the learning process.

Finding Reliable Resources: Establishing a Knowledge Foundation

A. Researching and identifying resources.

In the digital age, we have access to a variety of information. Beginners can benefit from exploring and choosing credible resources that align with their learning style. Whether it's books, online courses, video tutorials, or mentorship, using high-quality materials ensures a firm foundation and guided learning.

B. Seeking mentorship and guidance.

Mentorship is an invaluable resource for beginners. Connecting with experts in the subject delivers valuable insights, recommendations, and personalized assistance. Learning from someone who has faced similar issues can considerably speed up the learning process and provide practical insights that go beyond theoretical understanding.

Building Consistent Routine: The Habit of Practice

A. Prioritising Consistency over Intensity.

Consistency is essential in the early stages of any endeavour. Rather than occasional, strong bursts of work, adopting a regular and sustained habit promotes consistent improvement. Regular practice fosters habits, which, with time, contribute to skill and mastery.

B. Balancing the Quantity and Quality of Practice.

Finding the appropriate balance between quantity and quality of practice is critical. While regularity is important, making each practice session intentional and focused increases the effectiveness of learning. Quality practice entails deliberate attempts to improve abilities, comprehend concepts, and overcome specific problems.

Embracing Mistakes: Steps to Mastery

A. Redefining failure as feedback.

Mistakes are a normal part of the learning process. Instead of perceiving mistakes as failures, beginners can see them as important feedback. Each blunder provides insights into areas for progress and serves as a stepping stone to mastery. Embracing mistakes with a growth mentality promotes resilience and a positive outlook on obstacles.

B. Iterative Learning and Continuous Improvement

Learning is an iterative process. Beginners might adopt an iterative mentality, revising and enhancing their understanding or skills in response to feedback and experiences. Iterative learning is a cycle of experimenting, reflecting, and refining that allows for ongoing development and adaptation.

Effective Time Management: Maximising Learning Opportunities

A. Prioritising Learning Time

Time management is critical for beginners. Prioritizing learning time over other tasks ensures that progress is steady. Setting aside time for learning, even in little increments, accumulates over time and eliminates procrastination.

B. Balance Patience and Persistence

Learning takes time, and beginners may experience feelings of impatience. It is vital to strike a balance between patience and persistence. Recognizing that growth is a gradual process helps people stay committed to their journey, even when faced with obstacles.

Connecting with a Community: The Power of Support.

A. Joining Learning Communities

Engaging with a community of learners who share similar interests serves as a support system. Online forums, social media groups, and local gatherings provide opportunities to share ideas, seek assistance, and celebrate achievements. Connecting with a community develops feelings of belonging and encouragement.

B. Celebrating Progress Together.

Recognizing and enjoying little accomplishments is critical for beginners.

Every milestone, no matter how small, represents development and dedication. Sharing achievements with a group boosts motivation and reinforces a good attitude towards the learning process.

Reflection and Adaptation: A Dynamic Learning Process.

A. Reflecting on Progress and Challenges.

Regular self-reflection enables novices to evaluate their development and discover areas that want improvement. Reflecting on both triumphs and obstacles helps to have a better understanding of the learning process and guides strategic decisions.

B. Adaptability is a virtue.

Flexibility and adaptability are essential qualities in any learning process. As novices encounter new information, challenges, or developing goals, they must change their approach to ensure continuing growth. Embracing change and adapting techniques based on feedback helps to create a dynamic and resilient learning environment.

Asanas for Mental Clarity

In the labyrinth of modern life, where the rush and bustle sometimes dominate, finding moments of serenity and mental clarity becomes vital. The physical postures, or asanas, in yoga, not only shape the body but also serve as doorways to the mind.

Mind-Body Connection in Yoga

A. The Holistic Approach to Yoga

Yoga, which has its roots in ancient Indian philosophy, is a holistic approach that acknowledges the complex interplay between the body and mind. Physical postures, or asanas, are an essential component of yoga practice, aiming not just to improve physical flexibility and strength but also to foster mental clarity and inner serenity.

B. The Breath, Body, and Mind Trio

The relationship between the breath, body, and mind is central to yoga philosophy. When performed attentively, asanas synchronize with the breath, resulting in a dynamic interplay that teaches practitioners to stay present in the moment. The careful combination of breath and movement in asanas creates a meditation in action, promoting mental clarity by anchoring the mind to the rhythm of the breath.

Asanas for Mental Clarity: A Journey Within

A. Mountain Pose (Tadasana): Rooting in Stability.

The Mountain Pose, also known as Tadasana, is a basic position that promotes stability and balance. Standing tall with feet together, shoulders relaxed, and arms by their sides, practitioners ground themselves and connect with the earth beneath. Tadasana supports a focused gaze and a steady breath, instilling a sense of rootedness that extends to mental stability. This pose's simplicity makes it suitable for practitioners of all skill levels, offering a solid foundation for mental clarity.

B. Tree Pose (Vrikshasana) for Concentration

Vrikshasana, also known as Tree Pose, is a yoga posture in which you stand on one leg and place the other foot on your inner thigh or calf. Balancing in this stance demands concentration and mental focus. As practitioners achieve balance, the mind automatically quiets, providing a moment of peaceful mental clarity. Tree pose not only strengthens the legs and improves balance, but it also promotes mindfulness and inner quiet.

C. Downward-Facing Dog (Adho Mukha Svanasana): Calmness Through Inversion

Adho Mukha Svanasana, also known as Downward-Facing Dog, is an inversion with the head below the heart. This inversion increases blood flow to the brain, which promotes mental clarity and relaxation. As practitioners stretch their spine and press their heels to the floor, tension in the shoulders and neck is released, allowing for mental peace. Downward-Facing Dog is a dynamic pose that energizes the body and clears the mind.

D. Child's Pose (Balasana): Surrender to Inner Peace

Balasana (Child's Pose) is a restorative posture in which practitioners kneel, sit back on their heels, and fold forward with arms extended or resting by their sides. This soft forward bend promotes the surrender of the body and mind. As practitioners rest their foreheads on the mat, they experience inner calm and silence. Child's Pose promotes mental clarity by providing a moment of silence and submission.

E. Warrior II (Virabhadrasana II): Developing Strength and Focus.

Virabhadrasana II, or Warrior II, is a dynamic standing pose that strengthens the legs while opening the hips and chest. The extended arms and focused look on the front hand convey a sense of determination and concentration. This strong stance helps practitioners develop mental resilience and focus. Warrior II represents the warrior's unwavering focus on the way ahead, enabling practitioners to approach problems with clarity and strength.

F. Seated Forward Bend (Paschimottanasana): Relaxing the Mind

Paschimottanasana, also known as Seated Forward Bend, consists of sitting with legs extended and stretching forward to touch the toes. This mild forward fold stretches the spine and hamstrings while also relaxing the neurological system. As the practitioner softens into the pose, the breath deepens and the mind relaxes. Seated Forward Bend is a meditative pose that encourages introspection and mental focus.

Breath-Centric Asanas: Bridging the Physical and Mental .

A. Bridge Pose (Setu Bandhasana): Elevating with Breath

Setu Bandhasana, also known as Bridge Pose, entails raising the hips towards the sky while keeping the shoulders anchored. This backbend strengthens the spine and promotes deep breathing. The expansion of the chest and engagement of the core allows for deeper breaths, boosting mental clarity and rejuvenation. Bridge Pose acts as a link between the physical and mental realms, synchronizing breath with movement.

B. Cat-Cow Stretch (Marjaryasana-Bitilasana): Moving with Breath

The Cat-Cow Stretch is a dynamic movement that alternates between arching the back (Cow) and rounding the spine (Cat). This fluid movement, timed to the breath, improves spinal flexibility and relieves tension in the back and neck. The rhythmic pattern of Cat-Cow Stretch produces a moving meditation that promotes mental clarity by connecting breath and movement in a harmonious flow.

Corpse Pose (Savasana): Integrating the Practice

No discussion on yoga asanas for mental clarity is complete without including Savasana, or Corpse Pose. Savasana is a final resting pose in which practitioners lie on their backs and allow their bodies to fully relax. This asana completes the practice by merging the physical and mental benefits of the previous poses. Savasana induces great calm, resulting in a deep sensation of mental clarity and inner tranquility.

Flowing Through Yoga Sequences

Yoga sequences emerge as a dance of body and soul, with a delicate cadence of breath and movement. These sequences flow fluidly from one posture to the next, inviting practitioners to embark on a dynamic journey that goes beyond physical training and becomes a meditative discovery of self. In this article, we will delve into the essence of flowing through yoga sequences, examining the transforming impact of this practice in creating mind–body connection, balance, and a deep sense of presence.

The essence of yoga flow is a dance of breath and movement.

A. Understanding Vinyasa: Flowing Breath Connection

Vinyasa is a fundamental notion in flowing yoga sequences. Vinyasa describes the harmonious connection of breath and movement. In a vinyasa practice, each transition from one pose to the next is associated with a certain breath, resulting in a beautiful rhythm that elevates the entire practice. The synchrony of breath and movement converts the practice into a mindful meditation, fostering a higher level of awareness.

B. The Dynamic Dance of Asanas: Moving Meditation

Yoga sequences, also known as vinyasa flows, are a series of interconnected asanas intended to promote fluid, continuous movement. The practitioner gracefully transitions from one pose to the next, keeping a careful awareness of the breath throughout. This dynamic dance of asanas goes beyond the limitations of physical postures, enabling people to engage with their inner landscape of thoughts, sensations, and emotions.

Building Mind-Body Awareness with Yoga Sequences

A. Present Moment Awareness: At the Heart of Flowing Sequences

Flowing through yoga sequences promotes present-moment mindfulness. As practitioners move from posture to pose with intention and grace, they are urged to let go of past anxieties and future expectations. The constant flow encourages immersion in the present moment, developing a sense of mindfulness that transcends beyond the mat and into everyday life.

B. Tuning Into Sensations: A Mindful Investigation

Yoga sequences allow you to tune into your body's sensations. As participants move through the fluidity of postures, they are urged to watch the subtle alterations in muscle engagement, the breath's tempo, and the interaction of strength and flexibility. This increased sensory awareness opens the door to a better understanding of one's body and allows for self-discovery.

Transformative Power of Yoga Flow Sequences

A. Balanced Energy: The Dance of Opposites

Yoga sequences frequently include a combination of energizing and grounding postures. The dynamic interplay between backbends and forward folds, inversions, and grounding positions results in a dance of opposites. This balance not only improves physical health but also reflects the balance desired in the mental and emotional spheres. The ebb and flow of energy in the sequences harmonises the body's subtle energies, bringing balance and relaxation.

B. Developing Strength and Flexibility: A Symbiotic Relationship

The flowing quality of yoga sequences aids in the development of strength and flexibility. Each asana works in different muscle areas, increasing strength, while the continuous movement promotes flexibility. This mutually beneficial relationship between strength and flexibility not only improves physical performance but also reflects the interwoven nature of mental resilience and adaptation.

C. Emotional Release and Mindful Process

Yoga sequences serve as a container for emotional release and conscious processing. As practitioners progress through the sequences, they may confront physical challenges or discomfort. These experiences can act as doorways to emotional investigation. The conscious processing of emotions during the practice leads to a transformative journey of self-awareness and acceptance.

Crafting a Personal Flow: A Journey of Self-expression

A. Sequencing with Intention: Tailoring Practice

One of the benefits of flowing through yoga sequences is the ability to design a practice with purpose. Practitioners can select sequences that reflect their bodily demands, emotional emotions, or spiritual goals. Whether focused on heart-opening poses for emotional release or grounding poses for stability, the careful creation of sequences allows individuals to shape a practice that is unique to their path.

B. Finding Creative Expression: The Art of Flow.

Yoga routines may offer a platform for artistic expression. Practitioners can experiment with changes, transitions, and personal adjustments to the flow, allowing the practice to evolve as an art form. This creative expression not only brings delight to the practice but also represents the uniqueness of each practitioner's experience.

Mindfulness in Transition: Navigating Challenges Gracefully.

A. Presence in Transitions: The Heartbeat of Flow

The transitions between poses in yoga sequences are equally important as the poses themselves. Mindfulness in transitions entails staying connected to the breath and attentive while the body moves from one posture to the next. These transitional moments form a heartbeat inside the flow, allowing practitioners to traverse hurdles gracefully and with ease.

B. Adapting to Individual Needs: Respecting the Body

Flowing through yoga sequences helps practitioners to tailor the practice to their specific needs. This adaptability is a key component of mindful yoga. Honoring the body's signals, whether by changing poses for injury avoidance or adjusting the tempo based on energy levels, promotes self-care and compassion.

Cultivating a Meditative Mind: Stillness Within Movement.

A. Flow: Meditation in Motion.

Yoga sequences that seamlessly integrate breath and movement transform the practice into a moving meditation. As practitioners go through positions mindfully, their minds become absorbed in the rhythm of the breath and the dance of the body. The outside world recedes into the background, and a sensation of quiet occurs within the movement—a meditative state in which the mind finds peace.

B. Transcending Dualities: Unity in Flow.

The experience of flowing through yoga sequences transcends the distinction between mind and body. Practitioners experience a condition of integration in which the line between the physical and mental domains blurs. This transcendence develops a deep sense of unity, reminding people that yoga is more than just a physical practice; it is a holistic examination of oneself.

5

Chapter Four: Integrating Meditation and Yoga

Finding Harmony in Daily Life

Finding peace in today's maelstrom of responsibilities, demands, and constant connectedness can feel like a faraway echo. Yet, amid this maze, there lies a fundamental quest: a path toward balance, serenity, and inner peace.

Introduction: The Pursuit of Harmony in Chaos.

The quest for harmony in daily life is a tangible and transformational journey rather than a utopian ideal. It entails negotiating the obstacles of a fast-paced world while maintaining a strong connection with oneself and the environment. As we embark on this journey, let us peel back the layers of harmony, comprehend its essence, and discover practical techniques for incorporating balance and calm into our daily lives.

Understanding Harmony: A Multifaceted Symphony.

A. Balance the Elements of Life

Harmony in daily life is analogous to composing a symphony in which many elements—work, relationships, personal well-being, and leisure—flow together harmoniously. Harmony is achieved by recognizing these aspects' interconnectedness and consciously aligning them to produce a unified and melodic living experience.

B. Accepting the ebb and flow.

Harmony is not a static state, but rather a fluid dance of ebb and flow. It recognizes the inevitability of change and encourages people to embrace the rhythm of life with grace. Whether facing hardships or enjoying moments of joy, finding harmony necessitates an open-hearted understanding of life's ever-changing nature.

The Elements of Harmony: Balancing Work and Personal Life

A. Creating a Satisfying Work-Life Balance.

Work is an important part of daily life, and finding harmony entails striking a healthy work-life balance. This balance necessitates setting boundaries, prioritizing tasks, and acknowledging the value of rest and recreation. The goal is not only to divide time between business and personal life but to live each moment with intention and presence.

B. The Art of Presence: Quality Over Quantity.

Harmony is more than just how much time is spent in different facets of life; it is also about the quality of presence that is poured into those moments. Being fully engaged in the tasks at hand, whether at work or in personal contact, increases the richness of the experience. Mindfulness in daily tasks promotes a stronger connection to the present moment, resulting in a sense of harmony.

Cultivating Healthy Relationships: The Heart of Harmony

A. Communication and Connection.

Relationships are at the heart of daily life, and cultivating harmony within them requires good communication and true connection. Listening carefully, expressing thoughts and feelings openly, and cultivating empathy create a relational environment in which harmony can flourish. The quality of connections makes a substantial contribution to the overall harmony of daily exchanges.

B. Boundary and Mutual Respect

Harmonious partnerships demand healthy boundaries and mutual respect. Respecting individual needs, communicating expectations, and recognizing the value of personal space all help to create an environment in which relationships can thrive without jeopardizing individual well-being. This precise equilibrium forms the cornerstone of harmonious connections.

Self-care: Nurturing the Soul.

A. Prioritising Personal Wellbeing

Self-care, an often-overlooked discipline amid routine, is essential for everyday harmony. Prioritizing personal well-being entails deliberate actions of self-care, such as appropriate sleep, frequent exercise, and mindful eating. Spending time on things that bring joy and relaxation promotes a positive relationship with oneself.

B. Mind-Body Connection.

The mind and body are inextricably linked, and achieving balance necessitates nurturing the bond between them. Mindfulness meditation, yoga, and deep-breathing activities not only improve physical health but also help with mental clarity and emotional balance. The incorporation of mind-body activities into daily life creates a harmonizing energy that spreads beyond the individual to the surrounding environment.

Simplicity in Complexity: Streamlined Daily Tasks

A. The paradox of simplicity.

Amid the complexities of daily life, simplicity emerges as an effective ally in the pursuit of harmony. Simplifying daily duties entails clearing physical and mental space, prioritizing critical actions, and reducing superfluous complications. Embracing simplicity allows people to focus on what is genuinely important, creating a sense of ease and harmony.

B. Mindful Time Management.

Time is a valuable resource, and utilizing it carefully is critical to achieving harmony. Prioritizing work, setting realistic goals, and avoiding multitasking all help to improve time management. Adopting a thoughtful approach to time promotes a balanced distribution of energy, reduces stress, and improves overall harmony.

Nature and Mindful Reflection: Reconnecting to the Essence

A. The Healing Power of Nature

In the concrete jungles of everyday life, reconnecting with nature provides great harmony. Spending time outside, whether in a park, garden, or natural setting, provides a break from the stresses of urban life. Nature has a calming influence on the mind, allowing for introspection, renewal, and reconnection to life's underlying cycles.

B. Mindful Reflection Practices.

Harmony flourishes during periods of thoughtful reflection. Taking time for introspection, journaling, or engaging in contemplative practices assists people in obtaining insights into their values, goals, and life trajectories.

Mindful reflection serves as a compass, encouraging people to make decisions and take actions that are true to themselves.

Adaptability and Resilience: Managing Life's Changes

A. Accepting the impermanence of life

Harmony does not imply a lack of obstacles, but rather the ability to handle them with adaptability and perseverance. Embracing the impermanence of life is accepting that change is unavoidable and being willing to adjust to changing circumstances. This approach promotes resilience, helping people to accept problems with a sense of equilibrium and calm.

B. Learning from Challenges

Challenges are not hurdles to harmony, but rather chances for growth and learning. Each difficulty teaches significant lessons, and embracing them with a sense of inquiry and resilience turns adversity into a stepping stone to greater harmony. Learning from obstacles entails viewing setbacks as opportunities for personal and community growth.

Maximizing Benefits with Combined Practices

Individuals who seek holistic well-being and personal growth frequently experiment with a wide range of practices and methodologies. The goal of combining these approaches is not just to increase efficiency, but also to unleash synergies so that the sum becomes larger than the parts.

Introduction: The Interconnectedness of Well-Being

The human experience is multidimensional, including bodily health, mental clarity, emotional resilience, and spiritual fulfillment. As people navigate this complex landscape, they come across a diverse range of disciplines, including physical workouts, mindfulness techniques, and spiritual interests. The beauty is not just in the variety of these techniques, but also in the possible synergies that can develop when they interact.

Understanding the Power of Synergy

A. Beyond the Sum of Parts

Synergy, in the context of integrated activities, refers to the phenomenon in which the interplay of parts generates a result greater than the sum of their separate effects. It is the notion that some pairings magnify the benefits, resulting in a harmonious resonance that pervades all parts of one's existence.

B. Holistic well-being as the ultimate goal

The essence of combining disciplines is the quest for overall well-being. Rather than seeing physical health, mental well-being, and spiritual progress as separate spheres, people are recognising their interdependence. Maximizing advantages through combination practices acknowledges that true well-being occurs when diverse aspects of life are in balance.

Physical and Mindful Movement: A Dance of Body and Mind

A. Yoga and Mindfulness Exercise

The combination of yoga and mindful exercise shows the link between physical and mental health. Yoga, which focuses on breath awareness and mind-body connection, complements attentive workouts like walking, jogging, and even weight training. The result is a comprehensive approach to exercise that not only improves physical strength and flexibility but also promotes mental clarity and focus.

B. Tai Chi & Meditation

Tai Chi's slow, flowing movements, paired with meditation practices, produce a calming synergy that extends beyond physical activity. Tai Chi, also known as "meditation in motion," integrates breath, movement, and awareness. The combination of Tai Chi's beautiful postures and meditation increases the contemplative experience, encouraging relaxation, stress reduction, and improved mental health.

Mindfulness and Productivity: Cultivating Presence in Action

A. Mindful Work Practices

Combining mindfulness and work practices adds a transformative element to the working sphere. Mindful approaches to tasks, such as deep work, time management, and intentional breaks, improve focus and productivity. The incorporation of mindfulness into regular work routines promotes a work environment in which employees perform with greater awareness and efficiency.

B. Mindful Eating & Nutrition

Mindful eating practices are an example of how mindfulness and nutrition work together. Instead of hurrying through meals, people develop an awareness of the flavors, textures, and feelings connected with eating. This thoughtful approach not only encourages better food choices but also improves the overall dining experience, fostering a positive relationship with food.

Cultivating Emotional Intelligence: Mind-Heart Connection

A. Meditation for Emotional Resilience

Meditation, when combined with practices targeted at developing emotional intelligence, becomes an effective tool for emotional resilience. Mindful meditation, combined with strategies such as journaling or gratitude practices, allows people to navigate their emotions with better self-awareness. The end outcome is an emotional landscape marked by comprehension, acceptance, and a balanced approach to problems.

B. Artistic Expression and Emotional Release

The combination of artistic expression—whether through visual arts, music, or writing—and practices that focus on emotional well-being provides a cathartic release. Engaging in artistic endeavors allows for emotional expression and release. The combination of creativity and emotional processing creates a stronger connection with one's emotions and provides an outlet for self-discovery.

Spiritual Exploration and Mind-Body Practices: Aligning with the Soul

A. Meditation and Spiritual Connection

Meditation, which is frequently used to bridge the gap between the physical and spiritual realms, complements spiritual exploration. Individuals can strengthen their connection to their spiritual nature by practicing guided meditation, visualization, or transcendental meditation. The combination of meditation and spiritual activities results in a harmonic journey of self-discovery and transcendence.

B. Yoga & Mindful Spirituality

Yoga is more than just physical postures; it also includes a deliberate approach to spirituality. Combining yoga with spiritual activities like prayer or purposeful rituals results in a more comprehensive spiritual experience. The purposeful alignment of breath, movement, and spiritual attention fosters a relationship with the divine, resulting in inner calm and purpose.

The Importance of Intention: Creating a Purposeful Tapestry

A. Setting Intention for Combined Practices.

The key to optimizing benefits with combination approaches comes in having clear aims. Intentionality directs the focus of each activity and links it with larger aims. Whether the goal is stress relief, personal progress, or spiritual awakening, setting intentions ensures that each practice contributes meaningfully to the desired results.

B. Adapting Practices for Individual Needs

Every individual is unique, and the beauty of combination techniques stems from their versatility. Tailoring the combination of practices to individual requirements, tastes, and circumstances results in a more personalized approach to well-being. This versatility enables people to weave a tapestry of behaviors that reflect their true selves.

Overcoming Challenges: Navigating the Journey of Integration

A. Balancing time commitments.

One problem in combining practices is striking a balance between time obligations. However, the key is to prioritize and recognize that quality of contact is more important than quantity. Short, targeted practices incorporated into regular routines can be more lasting and effective than longer sessions.

B. Managing Overstimulation

Overstimulation is a widespread problem in today's information-rich society. Individuals can navigate this by taking a gradual approach, implementing one or two practices at a time. Mindful experimentation leads to a better understanding of the synergy between practices and their impact on general well-being.

6

Chapter FIVE: Advanced Practices

Deepening Meditation

I n the hectic fabric of modern life, when the outside world competes for attention, the journey within becomes a haven for the spirit. Meditation, an ancient practice that crosses cultural barriers, provides a path to profound self-discovery and inner calm.

Introduction: The Call to the Inner Sanctuary.

In a society full of nonstop action and commotion, the invitation to deepened meditation echoes like a whisper, asking people to focus their attention within. Meditation, which has its roots in several spiritual traditions, is a practice that transcends religious boundaries, providing a universal road to self-realization. The journey inside is not a retreat from the outside world, but rather a return to the essence of being—a sacred exploration of the inner landscape.

Understanding Deep Meditation: Beyond the Surface

A. Going Beyond the Surface Layers

Moving beyond the mind's superficial layers is necessary for deep meditation. Individuals must transcend the chatter of thoughts, the restlessness of emotions, and the continual stimulus of the outside world. As practitioners progress into the depths of meditation, they discover a stillness that is more than just the absence of noise, but also the presence of profound quietude.

B. Accepting the Present Moment

Deep meditation is fundamentally about embracing the present moment. Rather than concentrating on the past or projecting into the future, practitioners learn to stay present. This focused presence opens a portal to a timeless realm where the never-ending flow of thoughts gives way to a peaceful expanse of awareness.

The Foundations of Deepening Meditation: Breath and Awareness.

A. Breath as the Gateway to Presence.

The breath acts as an anchor in the sea of meditation. Deepening the breath becomes a deliberate act that corresponds to the rhythm of the present moment. Inhaling and exhaling become more than just physiological processes; they are a dance with the essence of existence. Focusing on the breath takes the mind's attention away from distractions and gently brings it into a state of calm.

B. Promoting Nonjudgmental Awareness

Deepening meditation entails developing nonjudgmental awareness—a state in which thoughts, sensations, and emotions are observed without attachment or aversion. Rather than categorizing events as positive or negative, practitioners approach them with curiosity and acceptance. This focused awareness provides inner space, allowing for a more in-depth connection with one's self.

Techniques for Deepening Meditation: An Exploration

A. Mindfulness meditation.

Mindfulness meditation, which originated in Buddhist traditions, is a commonly used approach for deepening meditation. It entails paying attention to the breath, bodily sensations, or the flow of thoughts without attachment. Mindfulness promotes non-reactive awareness, allowing people to watch mental changes with equanimity.

B. Loving-kindness Meditation

Loving-kindness Meditation, also known as Metta meditation, extends the practice of meditation beyond self-awareness. Practitioners create feelings of love and compassion for themselves, which they then transfer to others. This practice not only strengthens the inner connection but also promotes a sense of interconnection with all beings.

C. Body Scan Meditation.

Body scan meditation entails deliberately directing attention to various parts of the body to develop sensory awareness. This approach fosters a strong mind-body connection, allowing people to relieve tension and feel more at ease in both the physical and mental domains. The body becomes a portal into the current moment.

D. Transcendental Meditation.

Transcendental Meditation, popularised by Maharishi Mahesh Yogi, entails a quiet repetition of a mantra. This technique seeks to transcend regular thought and achieve a sublime state of pure consciousness. The mantra's repetition serves as a vehicle for transcending the mind's surface level and entering the depths of consciousness.

Deepening Meditation with Rituals and Environment

A: Creating a Sacred Space

Meditation's atmosphere has a huge impact on its depth. Creating a sacred space, whether it's a designated meditation room or a quiet area, encourages respect for the practice. The space's simplicity and tranquility facilitate the trip inward, signaling to the mind that it is time to enter a sacred realm.

B. Rituals & Preparatory Practices

Including rituals and preparatory practices in your meditation regimen creates a sense of continuity and intention. Lighting a candle, burning incense, or performing a quick grounding exercise creates a connection between the outside world and the contemplative environment. These rituals tell the mind that it's time to enter a state of deep presence.

Challenges to Deepening Meditation: Navigating the Inner Terrain

A. Mental restlessness and wanderings.

Restlessness and continuous mental wandering are common obstacles in deepening meditation. Rather than seeing these as impediments, practitioners are encouraged to approach them with patient curiosity. Each interruption serves as an opportunity to return the attention to the present moment, strengthening the meditation practice's resilience.

B. Impatience and Expectations.

Impatience and expectations frequently impede the process of deepening meditation. The trip within is not a linear path, but rather a dynamic inquiry with ebbs and flows. Cultivating patience and letting go of preconceived beliefs allows people to accept the unfolding nature of meditation, where each moment has its unique treasures.

Deepening Meditation: A Lifelong Journey

A: The Evolution of Practice

Deepening meditation is a never-ending journey. Individuals who practice meditation regularly experience the evolution of their inner environment. The practice becomes a mirror, reflecting the nuances of the mind, emotions, and an ever-deepening connection with oneself.

B. Incorporating Meditation into Daily Life.

The advantages of profound meditation extend beyond the cushion and into everyday life. Integrating mindfulness into ordinary tasks, such as walking, eating, or even working, expands the contemplative experience into everyday life. Mindfulness becomes a way of being, blurring the lines between meditation and ordinary living.

The Transformative Power of Deep Meditation

A. Enhancing Emotional Resilience.

Deepening meditation has a significant effect on emotional resiliency. The practice develops an awareness that transcends reactionary habits, allowing people to respond to emotions calmly. Emotional oscillations transform into a dance within the expanse of consciousness, promoting a healthy and resilient emotional landscape.

B. Promoting Clarity and Insight

Practitioners develop clarity and insight when the layers of their minds are gradually peeled away through deeper meditation. The meditative state provides a vantage point from which individuals can study thought patterns, the nature of desires, and the underlying reasons that drive their actions. This self-awareness serves as a guiding light as we navigate the intricacies of life.

Mastering Challenging Yoga Poses

The appeal of demanding poses in yoga draws practitioners into a transforming realm where physical power, mental focus, and spiritual connection all come together. The mastering of difficult yoga poses goes beyond the physical domain, into a profound exploration of one's capabilities, limitations, and the skill of fostering resilience.

Introduction: The Dance of Challenge and Growth.

Completing difficult yoga positions demonstrates the dynamic interplay between struggle and growth. These poses, also known as "asanas," push practitioners beyond their comfort zones, challenging them to overcome physical, mental, and occasionally emotional obstacles. The path to mastery is not about perfection, but rather a dance with the limits of capabilities, where each obstacle is an opportunity for growth.

Understanding Challenging Yoga Poses: Beyond the Surface.

A. Physical Complexity and Alignment.

Physical difficulty and meticulous alignment are what distinguish challenging yoga poses. These positions frequently need a combination of strength, flexibility, balance, and inversion. Examples of arm balances include the Crow Pose (Bakasana), inversions like Headstand (Sirsasana), and deep backbends like Wheel Pose (Urdhva Dhanurasana). Mastery of these poses necessitates a thorough understanding of body mechanics and alignment concepts.

B. Mental Focus and Mind-Body Connection.

Beyond physical prowess, achieving difficult yoga positions necessitates mental concentration and a stronger mind-body connection. The capacity to focus on the breath, retain present-moment awareness, and avoid mental distractions becomes critical. The process entails finding a balance between effort and surrender, where the mind helps the body navigate the complexities of each pose.

The Path to Mastery: Establishing Foundations

A. Building a Strong Foundation

The route to achieving difficult yoga poses begins with laying a solid foundation. This entails perfecting basic yoga positions to increase strength, flexibility, and body awareness. Poses such as Downward-Facing Dog (Adho Mukha Svanasana), Warrior Poses, and Plank serve as building blocks for the more complex tasks that lie ahead.

B. Gradual progression and patience.

Patience becomes a guiding partner on the journey to mastery. Practitioners often work their way up to more difficult poses by experimenting with different adjustments. Each step of the journey contributes to the process, allowing the body to gradually adapt, strengthen, and open. Cultivating patience becomes a practice in and of itself, cultivating an attitude of acceptance and patient persistence.

Breath as a Bridge: Managing Physical and Mental Challenges

A. Utilising the Power of Breath

The breath is a critical link in the route to learning difficult yoga positions. Conscious and controlled breathing not only provides oxygen to the body but also relaxes the mind. Integrating breath awareness into each pose generates a rhythmic flow that helps you retain attention, steadiness, and a sense of relaxation even in difficult postures.

B. Breath: A Tool for Mental Resilience

Challenging yoga positions frequently result in mental challenges, such as dread or self-doubt. The breath becomes a very useful tool for navigating various mental worlds. Practitioners learn to center themselves in the present moment by breathing steadily and intentionally, which reduces anxiety and promotes mental resilience.

Building Strength and Flexibility: The Physical Foundations

A. Targeted Strength-Building Exercises

Mastering difficult yoga poses necessitates focused strength in certain muscular regions. Strength-building workouts outside of regular yoga practice are necessary. Exercises like core strengthening, arm balances, and leg-focused routines help to establish the physical foundation required for advanced postures.

B. Progressional Flexibility Training

Flexibility is another essential component for mastering difficult poses. Progressive flexibility training, which includes both dynamic and static stretches, helps prepare the body for more difficult postures. Consistent and deliberate stretching, especially in the hips, hamstrings, and shoulders, improves the range of motion needed for advanced postures.

Mindful alignment and body awareness: the art of precision.

A. Alignment Principles: Guides

Mastering hard yoga poses necessitates a thorough understanding of alignment concepts. Each posture has distinct alignment clues that help practitioners achieve the best position for their bodies. Understanding the biomechanics and anatomical intricacies of each pose promotes both physical safety and a deeper connection to the pose's core.

B. Listening to Your Body's Feedback

Body awareness becomes an art on the path to mastery. Practitioners learn to listen to their bodies' subtle cues during each pose. Sensations of discomfort, tightness, or ease become essential clues for making modifications and maintaining a mindful approach to the practice. The key to mastering is to embody the pose with awareness and sensitivity, rather than just accomplishing it.

Advice from Experienced Teachers: A Supportive Framework

A. Seeking Knowledgeable Instruction.

The advice of experienced yoga teachers is crucial in the pursuit of mastering difficult positions. Knowledgeable instructors provide insights on pose mechanics, adjustments, and personalized instruction. Attending workshops, taking classes, and receiving individualized comments all contribute to a supportive environment that enhances the learning process.

B. Mentorship and Community Support.

Mentorship and community support are essential in the pursuit of mastery. Connecting with experienced practitioners, finding mentorship, and joining a supportive yoga group all bring encouragement, inspiration, and shared wisdom. The collective energy of a supportive community becomes a driving force on the path to achieving difficult poses.

Mind-body integration is the essence of mastery.

A. Developing Presence in Practice.

Mastery of difficult yoga positions goes beyond physical accomplishment; it represents the cultivation of presence. Practitioners learn to be present in each instant of their practice, immersing themselves in the experience without regard for the outcome. The voyage transforms into a meditative excursion, with the position serving as a gateway to the depths of inner consciousness.

B. Accepting the Learning Process

Mastery is a never-ending process of learning and improvement. Practitioners appreciate the beauty of the learning process, recognizing that each endeavor and difficulty contributes to personal growth. The poses become mirrors that reflect not only physical aptitude but also the resilience, patience, and self-awareness developed along the path.

Overcoming Fear and Building Confidence

A. Managing Fear Mindfully

Challenging yoga positions can elicit dread and self-doubt. Recognizing these emotions without judgment is essential for mindful fear navigation. Practitioners learn to recognize fear as a fleeting experience, acknowledging that it is a normal element of the transforming process. The breath becomes a form of anchoring, allowing people to navigate fear with grace.

B. Incremental Challenges to Confidence

Building confidence in tough poses requires a gradual escalation of obstacles. Practitioners can approach advanced poses with confidence by taking incremental steps built on a foundation of strength and alignment. Celebrating tiny triumphs along the way develops a positive attitude and increases confidence in one's abilities.

Incorporating Playfulness and Curiosity: Joy in Practice

A. Introducing Playfulness into Practice

Mastering difficult yoga positions is not without joy; it is a celebration of the joyful spirit. Incorporating playfulness into the practice entails investigating positions with interest, experimenting with variations, and taking a lighthearted approach. The trip transforms into an exploratory dance, with the pose serving as a happy expression of movement rather than a final destination.

B. Promoting Curiosity and Openness.

Cultivating curiosity entails always being open to new challenges. Practitioners avoid approaching positions with preconceived assumptions, instead remaining open to inquiry and discovery. Curiosity becomes a motivating drive that promotes exploration, adaptability, and the ongoing discovery of new dimensions within the practice.

Integrating Rest and Self-Care: Balancing Intensity

A. Recognise the Importance of Rest

The quest for mastery entails acknowledging the value of rest and rehabilitation. Challenging poses can put a strain on the body, therefore integrating recovery days into the practice program is essential. Rest permits the body to recover, avoiding burnout and promoting long-term success.

B. Self-care as a pillar of mastery.

Self-care is an essential component in the quest to achieve difficult yoga poses. It entails providing careful care for the body, such as massage, foam rolling, and proper sleep. Nurturing the body increases resilience, reduces damage, and promotes a balanced attitude to the practice.

Celebrating Progress: A Reflection on Mastery

A. Changing Focus from Perfection to Progress

Mastering difficult yoga poses requires shifting your focus from perfection to progress. Rather than focusing on reaching immaculate poses, practitioners applaud the gradual development made along the way. Each try, each improvement, represents a victory that reflects the growing mastery within.

B. Practicing Gratitude for the Journey

Gratitude becomes a guiding partner on the journey to mastery. Practitioners develop a respect for the path itself—the struggles, breakthroughs, and moments of self-discovery. The journey is transformed into a sacred pilgrimage, with each tough pose serving as a stepping stone to a better awareness of oneself.

Exploring Meditation Retreats and Yoga Workshops

In the middle of the hectic demands of modern life, there is a sanctuary for the soul—a place where people can escape the noise, reconnect with their inner selves, and go on transforming journeys. Meditation retreats and yoga workshops serve as entry points to these sacred spaces, providing immersive experiences that dig deeply into the worlds of mindfulness, self-discovery, and holistic wellness.

Introduction: The Cradle of Self-discovery

Meditation retreats and yoga workshops are more than just meetings; they are immersive experiences that aim to create a cocoon of reflection, healing, and renewal. In a world full of continual stimulation, these retreats and workshops provide pauses in time, inviting people to break aside from the exterior chaos and go on inner adventures.

Meditation retreats: the art of silence and stillness.

A. Accepting Silence as a Source of Power.

Meditation retreats frequently take place in calm areas surrounded by nature's tranquility. The practice of noble silence—an intentional moment of quiet in which participants refrain from verbal communication—is a defining feature of these retreats. Individuals who enjoy silence focus their attention inside, cultivating a deep connection with their thoughts, feelings, and the delicate subtleties of their inner world.

B. Immersive Meditation Practices.

The deep meditation practices that are incorporated throughout the daily agenda form the foundation of meditation retreats. Guided meditation sessions, mindfulness walks, and contemplative practices become essential components, moving people into higher levels of awareness. Individuals can meditate with heightened attention and a sensation of uninterrupted continuity in the retreat atmosphere, which is free of typical distractions.

C: Mindful Living and Conscious Awareness

Aside from traditional meditation sessions, meditation retreats emphasize mindful living as a comprehensive practice. Everyday actions like eating, walking, and even cleaning provide opportunities to develop conscious awareness. Participants learn how to incorporate mindfulness into many aspects of their lives, resulting in a smooth integration of meditation activities into daily routines.

D. Teacher Guidance and Spiritual Insight

Experienced meditation teachers frequently lead retreats, offering instruction and insights beyond basic meditation techniques. Philosophical talks, thoughts on mindfulness in daily life, and the investigation of spiritual notions are all possible topics for the training. On the inner journey, the instructor serves as both an inspiration and a guide.

Yoga Workshops: Dynamic Flow of Body and Spirit

A. Dynamic Asana Practices.

Yoga workshops, on the other hand, are lively gatherings that concentrate on the physical side of the practice—the asanas, or yoga postures. These seminars, guided by qualified instructors, explore the intricacies of alignment, breath, and energy flow inside the body. Participants complete a series of carefully chosen asanas to test the breadth and depth of their physical ability.

B. Investigating the Breath-Movement Connection

The investigation of the breath-movement relationship is an essential component of yoga workshops. Participants learn to synchronize their breath with each action, resulting in a dance-like flow. Conscious breathing not only improves physical practice but also opens the door to building awareness and presence on the mat.

C. Deepening Yogic Philosophy.

While yoga seminars primarily focus on physical practice, they frequently incorporate yogic philosophy. Instructors may incorporate discussions about the Eight Limbs of Yoga, the philosophy of non-attachment (Aparigraha), and the concept of attaining balance (Sthira and Sukha) into the workshop's fabric. This integration deepens the physical practice by inviting participants to connect with the spiritual underpinnings of yoga.

D. Community and Shared Energy

Yoga programs thrive on the combined energy of the attendees. The shared space becomes a community in which people support and encourage one another in their practice. The synergy established in these seminars develops a sense of community, improving the whole experience and frequently resulting in connections that continue beyond the mat.

Choosing the Right Experience: Things to Consider

A. Personal goals and intentions.

Personal objectives and intentions typically determine whether to attend a meditation retreat or a yoga session. If the goal is to deepen meditation techniques, investigate inner calm, and embrace silence, a meditation retreat may be the best option. A yoga workshop, on the other hand, would better align with the goals of refining physical postures, increasing flexibility, and exploring the physical aspects of yoga.

B. Preferred Learning Style.

When deciding between a meditation retreat and a yoga class, one should keep their preferred learning approach in mind. If an individual prefers the quiet and introspective components of learning, a meditation retreat may be a better fit. Yoga workshops may be more appealing to those who enjoy dynamic, physical interaction and hands-on learning experiences.

C. Level of Experience and Comfort

The level of familiarity and comfort with the methods available in each context is an important consideration. Meditation retreats frequently cater to practitioners of all levels, including novices, and offer a friendly setting for those new to meditation. Yoga seminars can vary in intensity, with some geared for beginners and others for more advanced practitioners. Choosing an experience appropriate for one's present level offers a positive and fulfilling immersion.

D. Duration and Commitment.

Meditation retreats and yoga workshops occur in a variety of lengths, from weekend retreats to prolonged immersions. Consideration of time commitment and availability is critical. A shorter workshop may be better suited to people with limited time, whilst longer retreats provide a more immersive experience and allow for a deeper dig into the practices.

Benefits of Retreats and Workshops: A Holistic View

A. Increasing self-awareness.

Meditation retreats and yoga courses both help people become more aware of themselves. Individuals gain insight into their thought patterns, emotional responses, and physical experiences by engaging in focused practices. The reflecting character of these experiences allows for self-discovery and a greater knowledge of the interdependence of mind, body, and spirit.

B. Stress Reduction & Relaxation

Retreats and workshops provide a break from the stresses of everyday life. The purposeful practice of mindfulness, whether through meditation or yoga, improves relaxation and stress reduction. Participants frequently leave these encounters with a restored sense of peace and the ability to use this tranquility in their daily lives.

C. Physical and Mental Wellbeing

The physical practices in yoga programs help to improve physical well-being. Common results include improved flexibility, strength, and posture. Meditation retreats, on the other hand, have a substantial positive impact on mental health by promoting mental clarity, emotional resilience, and inner serenity. These behaviors work together to promote overall well-being.

D. Connection and Community.

Both settings encourage connection and community. Participants frequently feel a sense of belonging, whether on a meditation retreat or at a yoga course. The collaborative nature of these events creates a conducive setting for personal development and shared exploration.

Challenges and Considerations: Navigating the Inner Landscape.

A. Potential Discomfort from Silence

Meditation retreats, particularly ones emphasizing noble silence, may cause discomfort for people who are not accustomed to long periods of stillness. The difficulty is to embrace the discomfort as part of the transformational process, enabling the mind to settle into quiet.

B. Physical Intensity at Yoga Workshops

Yoga seminars, especially those meant for advanced practitioners, may be physically demanding. The intensity of the practice might push people past their apparent boundaries. Listening to the body, talking with teachers, and maintaining personal limits are all necessary for navigating these issues.

C. Integrating Insights into Daily Life

Integrating insights into daily life is a common problem following retreats and workshops. Participants may return to the demands of their routines, and the goal is to discover methods to incorporate the mindfulness and self-awareness developed during these experiences into daily actions and decisions.

D. Managing Expectations.

Expectations influence the overall experience. Managing expectations entails acknowledging that these retreats and seminars are not miracle cures, but rather catalysts for personal growth. Participants may face problems, frustrations, or revelations, and accepting these features as part of the journey improves the entire experience.

Chapter Six: Overcoming Obstacles

Addressing Common Misconceptions

In the tapestry of human understanding, certain disciplines, such as meditation and yoga, have weaved old wisdom into the fabric of modern existence. However, as these transformative disciplines gain popularity, misconceptions have emerged, obscuring the profound truths that lie therein.

Introduction: Navigating the Landscape of Misconception

Meditation and yoga, which have their origins in several cultural traditions, have gained popularity worldwide in recent decades. However, their growing popularity has resulted in a variety of myths, fostered by a combination of cultural misinterpretations, sensationalism, and oversimplification. Addressing these misconceptions is critical for revealing the depth and authenticity that underpin these ancient practices.

Misconception 1: Meditation involves emptying the mind.

Reality: cultivating awareness, not emptiness.

One common misperception regarding meditation is that practitioners must clear their brains of all thoughts. In truth, meditation is about increasing awareness and presence rather than reaching mental emptiness. It entails watching thoughts without connection, allowing them to come and go like clouds. The emphasis is on developing a relationship with the mind rather than pursuing an impossible emptiness.

Misconception 2: Yoga is Only Physical Exercise.

Reality: The Union of Mind, Body, and Spirit

A prevalent misconception is that yoga is only a form of physical exercise. While the physical postures, or asanas, are a visible feature of yoga, they are only one component of the larger system established in ancient yogic philosophy. Yoga is a comprehensive practice that combines physical postures, breath control (pranayama), ethical precepts (yamas and niyamas), and meditation to promote the integration of mind, body, and spirit.

Misconception 3: You must be flexible to practice yoga.

Reality: Yoga is for Everybody.

The assumption that one must be extremely flexible to practice yoga is a common myth that precludes many potential practitioners. In reality, yoga is accessible and adaptable to all body shapes and levels of flexibility. The essence of yoga is the journey of self-discovery and self-care, not the ability to perform contortionist-like poses. Props and modifications are encouraged in yoga to make the practice more accessible to everyone.

Misconception 4: Meditation Requires a Quiet Mind

Reality: Accepting the Mind's Nature

Expecting a completely peaceful mind during meditation is a common myth that discourages newcomers. Meditation is not about suppressing thoughts, as the mind is designed to generate them. Instead, it emphasizes a peaceful, nonjudgmental observation of thoughts. Accepting the ebb and flow of thoughts is an essential element of the meditation process since it fosters a caring relationship with the mind.

Misconception 5: Yoga is a religion.

Reality: A Spiritual Practice, not a Religion.

Associating yoga with a certain religion, notably Hinduism, is a fallacy that obscures its universality. Yoga has its roots in ancient Indian philosophy, but it transcends religion. Yoga is a spiritual discipline that encourages people to explore their inner landscapes and connect with universal parts of consciousness. It can be used in conjunction with other religious beliefs or as a secular activity.

Misconception 6: Meditation requires sitting cross-legged.

Reality: Different meditation postures exist.

The idea of cross-legged meditation is profoundly embedded in popular culture, although it is not the only method of meditation. There are various meditation postures available, and people can choose whichever seems most comfortable to them. Sitting in a chair, kneeling, or even lying down are all suitable meditation postures. The aim is to establish a position that allows for both awareness and relaxation, resulting in a more sustainable and enjoyable practice.

Misconception 7: Meditation and Yoga are time-consuming practices.

Reality: Adapting Practices to Fit Life

The idea that meditation and yoga require considerable time commitments can turn off potential practitioners. In actuality, both techniques can be tailored to fit individual schedules. Short, steady sessions can be just as effective as longer ones. Integrating mindfulness into daily activities and short yoga sequences into routines can make these practices more accessible and sustainable.

Misconception 8: You need a certain space to meditate.

Reality: Create Mindful Moments Anywhere

Believing that meditation necessitates a dedicated, peaceful environment is a misconception that limits the practice's versatility. While having a dedicated meditation room can be useful, meditation is adaptable to a variety of settings. It can be practiced in a quiet room, during a lunch break at work, or even outdoors. The key is to cultivate a conscious mentality instead of relying only on external conditions.

Misconception 9: Yoga is only for the young and fit.

Reality: Yoga is inclusive of all ages and abilities.

A common fallacy is that yoga is only for the young, flexible, and physically fit. Yoga is truly inclusive, and it can be tailored to people of all ages, body kinds, and abilities. Specialized classes are designed for seniors, people with physical impairments, and those looking for gentle or restorative techniques. Yoga's versatility makes it suitable for people at all phases of life.

Misconception 10: Meditation and Yoga are quick fixes for mental health issues.

Reality: Complementary Practices for Mental Wellbeing

It is a common misconception that meditation and yoga can provide instant relief for mental health issues. While these activities have significant advantages for mental health, they are not fast cures. They necessitate persistent and thoughtful engagement throughout time. Meditation and yoga can be beneficial components of a comprehensive approach to mental health, but they should be supplemented with expert supervision as needed.

Overcoming Misconceptions: A Journey of Discovery

Addressing misconceptions about meditation and yoga entails dispelling myths and accepting the practices' validity. It is a journey of discovery and comprehension that defies popular stereotypes. Practitioners and individuals interested in these fields are encouraged to approach them with an open mind, allowing their unique experiences and discoveries to develop their knowledge.

Approaching the Path with Openness and Curiosity

Individuals who embark on the disciplines of meditation and yoga benefit greatly from an open and curious mindset. Rather than clinging to preconceived assumptions, accepting the mobility of these techniques provides for a more true and transforming experience. Meditation and yoga, when addressed with an open heart and a willingness to learn, reveal themselves to be ageless instruments for self-discovery, overall well-being, and a deeper connection with life's deepest mysteries.

Troubleshooting Challenges in Consistency

Consistency emerges as a key to achieving personal and professional goals, connecting ideas with tangible outcomes. However, the quest to retain consistency is frequently marked by peaks and valleys, as well as unexpected hurdles that might interrupt the regular rhythm of growth.

Introduction: The Dynamic Nature of Consistency.

Consistency, defined as the firm commitment to a specific method of doing things, is a driving force that propels people towards their goals. Whether pursuing physical objectives, professional advancements, or personal development, the ability to sustain consistency turns aspirations into tangible results. However, the path to consistency is far from straightforward, as it encounters a slew of obstacles that put one's resolve and adaptability to the test.

The Common Challenges in Consistency: Unveil the Obstacles

1. Motivational Peaks and Valleys

- **Challenge:** Motivation, the motivating force behind constant efforts, frequently fluctuates. Individuals with high drive can achieve extraordinary things, whereas those with low motivation may procrastinate and lack passion for long-term work.
- **Troubleshooting**: Increase intrinsic motivation by linking behaviors to personal beliefs and long-term objectives. Break down major goals into smaller, more manageable chores to keep you motivated even when you're feeling low.

2. Overcoming Procrastination

- **Challenge:** Procrastination, the delay of chores or goals, is a common difficulty that hinders consistency. It is generally caused by a combination of dread, hesitation, or a perception of the task's complexity.
- **Troubleshooting:** Divide tasks into smaller, more doable chunks. Use time management strategies, set deadlines, and create a setting that reduces distractions. Recognize and address the underlying reasons for procrastination to cultivate a proactive mindset.

3. Unforeseen Life Events

- **Challenge:** Unexpected events like health concerns, family emergencies, or professional pressures can interrupt patterns and make consistency difficult.
- **Troubleshooting:** Be flexible while creating goals. Create backup plans for disruptions and practice self-compassion in difficult situations. Maintain a sense of balance and adjust to changing situations.

4. Inadequate Planning

- **Challenge**: Uncertainty can hinder consistent efforts. Individuals without a defined plan may struggle to efficiently prioritize work.
- **Troubleshooting:** Develop a clear plan that includes explicit, quantifiable, and attainable targets. Break down huge goals into actionable actions with attainable dates. Regularly review and revise the strategy as needed to guarantee its relevance and alignment with changing priorities.

5. Burnout and Exhaustion

- **Challenge:** Excessive exertion might cause burnout. Exhaustion, both physical and mental, can lead to a loss of motivation and make it difficult to maintain desirable levels of consistency.
- **Troubleshooting:** Use smart breaks and self-care techniques to avoid burnout. Recognize indicators of weariness and modify the intensity

and length of your activities accordingly. Prioritise rest, relaxation, and rejuvenating activities for both the body and mind.

6. Lack of Accountability

- **Challenge:** Without external or internal accountability, individuals may struggle to stay on course. The lack of a support structure can undermine the commitment to consistent action.
- **Troubleshooting:** Create accountability frameworks by sharing goals with a trusted buddy, joining a community with similar aims, or engaging a coach. Regularly monitor progress and praise accomplishments to instill a sense of accountability in oneself.

Strategies to Improve Consistency: Building Resilience and Adaptability.

1. Develop intrinsic motivation: Intrinsic motivation, which is based on personal beliefs and real interest, acts as a stabilizing factor that can tolerate oscillations. Connect goals to significant values, appreciate modest triumphs, and cultivate a feeling of purpose to motivate ongoing efforts.

2. Prioritise: Goal Clarity and Planning: Clear, well-defined objectives and structured plans create a road map for consistent action. Break down goals into manageable steps, establish realistic timelines, and reassess and adjust plans regularly to reflect changing priorities.

3. Embrace flexibility and adaptability: Consistency does not indicate rigidity; rather, it promotes adaptation. Accept the truth of life's unpredictability and be prepared to change plans if unexpected obstacles arise. Developing resilience and flexibility enables long-term consistency.

4. Establish accountability structures: External and internal accountability measures ensure consistency. Share your goals with a trusted friend, join a supportive community, or seek the guidance of a mentor or coach. Regularly evaluate progress, consider problems, and alter plans as appropriate.

5. Prioritise self-care and balance: Consistent effort necessitates a sense of well-being. Prioritise self-care habits such as getting enough sleep, eating well, and exercising regularly. Strike a balance between work and recreation, understanding that long-term stability comes from a comprehensive approach to health.

6. Learn from setbacks and celebrate progress: View setbacks as chances for learning and progress, rather than failures. Reflect on challenges, discover lessons, and modify strategies accordingly. Celebrate progress, no matter how minor, to maintain a good outlook and motivation.

7. Establish routines and rituals: Routines and rituals typically promote consistency. Developing daily or weekly habits lays the groundwork for long-term success. Rituals work as cues for the brain, signaling the beginning and completion of specific activities and instilling a sense of predictability.

8. Seek support and collaboration: Consistency does not have to be an alone path. Seek encouragement from friends, family, or coworkers who share your aspirations. Collaboration can bring incentive, accountability, and a common feeling of accomplishment.

8

Chapter Seven:Tailoring Practices to Your Lifestyle

Quick Sessions for Busy Days

Maintaining a consistent wellness routine can be difficult in today's fast-paced world, where time frequently feels like a scarce resource. Work, family, and daily commitments might make it difficult to devote time to self-care. However, in the face of these constraints, there is a potent solution: brief sessions designed to incorporate moments of well-being into even the busiest days .

Introduction: The Pace of Modern Life

As our lives become more hectic, making time for self-care might feel like a luxury. The pressure of deadlines, family obligations, and the constant juggling act of everyday chores frequently push personal well-being to the sidelines. However, in the middle of the chaos, the need to carve out time for self-care routines grows even stronger. Quick workouts adapted for busy days emerge as beacons of balance, delivering a breather from the hectic pace while ensuring that wellness remains a priority.

Understanding the Need for Quick Sessions.

1. Time Constraints:

- **Challenge**: The main challenge is the limited amount of time available. The traditional concept of long workouts or extensive meditation periods may appear incompatible with hectic schedules.
- **Solution:** Quick sessions address this issue immediately, giving an easy entrance point into wellness without requiring a substantial time investment.

2. Mental tiredness:

- **Challenge:** Busy days can cause mental tiredness, making engaging in demanding activities less appealing.
- **Solution:** Short, targeted sessions are intended to be energizing rather than taxing, providing a mental break without adding to the day's workload.

3. Struggles with Consistency:

- **Challenge:** It can be challenging to establish and maintain a consistent program when long sessions are not feasible.
- **Solution:** Quick sessions promote consistency by adapting to daily schedule changes, allowing individuals to smoothly integrate wellness into their routines.

Anatomy of Quick Sessions: Tailoring Wellness for Busy Lives

1. Micro-Workouts for Physical Vitality.

.Quick Cardio Bursts:

- ***Routine***: Quick cardio bursts involve high-intensity workouts such as jumping jacks, high knees, and sprints.
- ***Impact:*** Increases heart rate, metabolism, and energy levels.

.5 Minute Strength Circuits:

- ***Routine***: Perform compound exercises such as squats, lunges, and push-ups in fast succession.
- ***Impact:*** Targets several muscular areas, increasing strength and toning.

.Express Yoga Flows:

- ***Routine:*** Express Yoga Flows are fast-paced routines that emphasize dynamic poses and movements.
- ***Impact:*** Improves flexibility, and posture, and gives a peaceful mental break.

2. Mindfulness in Minutes:

. Mini Meditation Breaks:

- ***Routine***: Short mindfulness meditation sessions focused on breath aware-ness or guided meditation.
- ***Impact:*** Reduces tension, improves mental clarity, and promotes a state of calm.

.Mindful Resets:

- *Routine:* Take a minute to observe your surroundings and focus on your senses.
- *Impact:* Keeps people grounded in the present moment, encouraging attention amid busyness.

.Breathwork Breaks:

- *Routine:* Quick sessions of intentional breathing exercises, such as deep diaphragmatic breathing.
- *Impact:* Relaxes the neurological system, relieves tension, and offers a mental reset.

3. Efficient Nutrition Practices:

.Smart Snacking:

- *Routine:* Prepare quick, nutrient-dense snacks such as nuts, yogurt with berries, or smoothies.
- *Impact:* Promotes continuous energy, satisfies appetite, and nourishes the body.

.Hydration Focus:

- *Routine:* To focus on hydration, create a routine that includes frequent water intake throughout the day.
- *Impact:* Promotes general health, improves digestion, and reduces weariness.

4. Refreshing Mental Breaks:

.Nature Connections:

- *Routine:* Take short walks or spend time in nature, even if only for a few minutes.

- **Impact:** Refreshes the mind, relieves mental weariness, and improves overall well-being.

.Creativity Breaks:

- *Routine:* Creativity breaks involve routinely engaging in creative activities such as sketching, writing, or listening to music.
- *Impact:* Encourages creativity, provides a mental break, and creates a sense of happiness.

Benefits of Quick Sessions: A Holistic Perspective

1. Physical Wellbeing:

- **Efficient Fitness:** Quick workouts help to preserve physical vitality by improving cardiovascular health, muscle tone, and flexibility.
- **Energy Boost:** Engaging in short, exhilarating activities can boost energy levels, battle exhaustion, and promote overall health.

2. Mental Health:

- **Stress Reduction:** Mindfulness and relaxation activities can reduce stress and improve mental clarity.
- **Improved Focus:** Taking quick mental breaks improves cognitive function, which supports increased focus and productivity.

3. Developing Consistency and Habits:

- **Adaptable Routine:** Quick sessions can fit daily schedule changes, making consistency easier to achieve.
- **Establishing behaviors:** The convenience of implementing brief sessions promotes the development of long-term wellness behaviors.

4. Emotional Wellness:

- **Mood Enhancement:** Endorphins are released by physical activity and mindfulness techniques, which enhance mood.
- **Stress Coping Mechanism:** Quick sessions are excellent stress-reduction strategies that promote emotional resilience.

5. Time Efficiency:

- **Optimal Use of Time:** Quick sessions maximize the efficient use of time, making wellness accessible even during the busiest days.
- **Integration into Daily Life:** Short breaks blend seamlessly into regular activities, ensuring that wellbeing is a part of everyday

Integrating Quick Sessions into Busy Days: A Personal Approach

1. Prioritising Self-Care:

- **Mindset Shift:** Making self-care a top priority regardless of time restrictions.
- **Setting Boundaries:** Creating clear boundaries to protect scheduled self-care time during the day.

2. Establishing a Personalised Routine:

- **Identifying preferences:** Choosing activities that are personally meaningful to ensure happiness and long-term participation.
- **range and Adaptability:** Including a range of short sessions to avoid monotony and altering routines to meet changing preferences.

3. Integrate Mindful Breaks Strategically:

- **Strategic Integration:** Plan small health breaks throughout the day.

- **Utilizing Breaks:** Taking advantage of short breaks during work or daily responsibilities for a fast session.

4. Leveraging Technology:

- **Guided Sessions:** Use applications or online tools for guided workouts, meditation, or mindfulness sessions.
- **Scheduled Reminders:** Setting reminders on devices to promote wellness-focused times.

5. Fostering Accountability:

- **Accountability Partners:** Partner with friends, family, or colleagues to discuss wellness objectives and encourage one other.
- **Celebrating Success:** Recognise and celebrate consistent accomplishments, no matter how minor.

Adapting for Various Fitness Levels

In the kaleidoscope of fitness, inclusion stands out as a fundamental value that transcends age, skill, and experience. Adapting workouts to accommodate different fitness levels emerges as a key component in creating a culture of accessibility and empowerment in the field of physical well-being.

Introduction: Beyond One Size Fits All.

In the vivid tapestry of fitness, the concept of a one-size-fits-all approach is gradually giving way to a more nuanced understanding—a recognition that each person embarks on a unique fitness path molded by personal goals, physical skills, and preferences. Recognizing and modifying routines for different fitness levels is more than simply a matter of practicality; it demonstrates the inclusive spirit that characterizes a holistic approach to health and wellness.

Understanding Different Fitness Levels.

1. Novices and Beginners:

- **Characteristics:** Limited familiarity with training, reduced baseline fitness, and possibly fear.
- **Adaptations:** Focus on fundamental movements, progressive advancement, and confidence building through attainable tasks.

2. Intermediate Levels:

- **Requirements**: Moderate fitness, experience with fundamental exercises, and desire for higher intensity.
- **Adaptations:** Introducing new exercises, integrating resistance training, and emphasizing progressive overload to ensure sustained improvement.

3. Advanced Fitness Enthusiasts:

- **Requirements:** high fitness proficiency, consistent training history, and a passion for demanding and diverse workouts.
- **Adaptations:** Advanced routines, higher-intensity intervals, and personalized programming to meet specific fitness goals.

4. Older Adults:

- **Characteristics:** Varied fitness levels, potential mobility or joint considerations, and a focus on maintaining overall health.

- **Adaptations:** low-impact workouts, functional motions, and adjustments to meet age-related problems.

5. Individuals with Health Conditions:

- **Characteristics:** Different fitness levels, medical concerns, and need for specialized assistance.
- **Adaptations:** customizing activities to fit unique health issues, emphasizing safety, and working with healthcare specialists.

The Importance of Adaptation in Fitness: A Comprehensive View

1. Accessibility and inclusivity:

- **Breaking barriers:** Adapting routines makes fitness accessible to people of all ages, body kinds, and abilities, establishing a culture of inclusivity.
- **Promoting longevity:** A personalized strategy promotes long-term involvement and a lifetime commitment to physical well-being.

2. Individualised Progression:

- **Empowering Journeys:** Recognising and adjusting to varied fitness levels allows individuals to improve at their own pace and feel a sense of accomplishment.
- **Sustainable Motivation:** Personalised adaptations help to maintain motivation by aligning workouts with personal goals and aspirations.

3. Building Confidence:

- **Celebrating Achievements:** Tailoring workouts promotes accomplishment and builds confidence in fitness journeys.
- **Overcoming Challenges:** Adapting exercises assist individuals in navigating adversities, fostering a sense of resilience and tenacity.

4. Injury Prevention and Longevity:

- **Mindful Programming:** Adaptations consider potential vulnerabilities, reducing the risk of injuries and promoting long-term health.
- **Increasing Consistency:** By reducing the chance of injury, adaptations help to maintain consistency in workout programs.

5. Addressing Diverse Goals:

- **Goal Alignment:** Adaptations tailor workouts to specific objectives, such as weight loss, muscle gain, or improved health.
- **Personalized Journey:** Recognising different fitness levels allows for personalized fitness journeys, which fosters a sense of ownership and dedication.

Adapting Workouts for Different Fitness Levels: Practical Considerations

1. Tailoring Intensity:

- **Beginners:** Start with low to moderate intensity, gradually increasing as fitness improves.
- **Intermediates**: Use a combination of moderate and high-intensity intervals to encourage improvement.
- **Advanced**: Challenge with high-intensity workouts, utilizing advanced methods and variations.

2. Exercise Modifications:

- **Beginners:** Focus on foundational movements with modifications as needed (e.g., knee push-ups instead of standard push-ups).
- **Intermediates:** Introduce variations and progressions (e.g., plank variations, adding resistance).

- **Advanced:** Include sophisticated movements and variations (e.g., plyometric workouts, advanced yoga positions).

3. Customizing Reps and Sets:

- **Beginners:** Start with lower reps and sets, gradually increasing as endurance improves.
- **Intermediates:** Include moderate rep and set ranges, emphasizing controlled form.
- **Advanced:** Increase the reps and sets to allow for progressive overload and muscle adaptation.

4. Prioritizing Recovery:

- **Beginners:** Emphasize adequate rest between exercises and sessions, prioritizing recovery.
- **Intermediates:** Use active recovery strategies and try varying workout intensities.
- **Advanced:** Use targeted recovery tactics such mobility exercises, stretching, and recovery-focused sessions.

5. Individualized Programming:

- **Beginners:** Focus on foundational movements, with an emphasis on form and technique.
- **Intermediates:** Increase workout diversity and development while keeping individual goals in mind.
- **Advanced:** Create personalized programs that are connected with specific fitness goals, including periodization for best outcomes.

Creating Inclusive Fitness Environments: From Gyms to Virtual Spaces

1. Gym Settings:

- **Qualified Instructors:** Gyms should employ qualified instructors who are skilled in adapting workouts for various fitness levels.
- **Diverse Class Offerings:** Offer a variety of classes for all fitness levels, from beginning to advanced.
- **Encouragement Environment:** Create a friendly and inclusive environment in which people feel comfortable tailoring workouts to their needs.

2. Virtual Fitness Platforms:

- **Varied Workout Options:** Virtual platforms should offer a diverse array of workout options, clearly labeled for different fitness levels.
- **Interactive Support:** Include tools such as live chats or forums where users can get guidance on how to modify activities.
- **Progress Tracking:** Give users tools to measure their progress and celebrate milestones, instilling a sense of accomplishment.

3. Community Engagement:

- **Community Events:** Organize fitness events that encourage participation from individuals of all fitness levels.
- **Online Communities:** Create online forums for people to discuss their experiences, challenges, and adjustments, generating a sense of community.

Success Stories: Understanding the Impact of Adaptation

1. Personalised Transformations:

- **Beginners:** Celebrate individuals who started with basic exercises and gradually progressed, achieving notable transformations.
- **Intermediates:** Share success stories from those who changed their routines to meet specific goals, demonstrating progression.
- **Advanced:** Feature people who completed advanced training regimens, emphasizing the transforming effect on their fitness.

2. Overcoming hurdles:

- **Beginners:** Share narratives of individuals who overcame initial challenges, inspiring others to embark on their fitness journey.
- **Intermediates:** Share experiences of tenacity in the face of plateaus, showcasing the power of adaptation and evolution.
- **Advanced:** Highlight athletes or fitness enthusiasts who have overcome difficult hurdles, inspiring others to push their limits.

3. Inclusive Fitness Communities:

- **Celebrating Diversity:** Showcase the diversity within fitness communities, featuring individuals from various age groups, backgrounds, and fitness levels.
- **Supportive Networks:** Emphasise the importance of supportive communities in motivating people to modify their exercises and attain their goals.

9

Chapter Eight:Sustaining a Lifelong Practice

Building a Supportive Community

I n the rich tapestry of personal well-being, the thread of community weaves a story of shared goals, encouragement, and development. A supportive community is more than just a group of people; it is a moving force that empowers, inspires, and develops a sense of belonging.

Introduction: The Essence of Supportive Community

In the world of well-being, the importance of community goes far beyond the physical act of being near others. A supportive community is an ecosystem where people get together not only to discuss exercise regimens or nutritional suggestions, but also to offer encouragement, celebrate accomplishments, and find solace during difficult times. It is a collaborative journey in which the sum of shared experiences weaves a tapestry of understanding, empathy, and shared accomplishments.

Foundations of a Supportive Community

1. Fostering Empathy and Understanding:

- **Creating Safe Spaces:** Create a safe place where individuals can share their weaknesses, problems, and triumphs without judgment.
- **Active Listening:** Create a culture of active listening to ensure that community members feel heard and understood.

2. Encouraging Inclusivity:

- **Diversity and Inclusion:** Create an inclusive workplace that embraces people from different backgrounds, fitness levels, and wellness aspirations.
- **Celebrating Differences:** Celebrate the community's variety, including each member's unique journeys and opinions.

3. Shared Accountability:

- **Mutual Support:** Encourage positive support and accountability among members.
- **Goal Sharing**: Create an environment in which people feel comfortable discussing their wellness objectives, resulting in a collective sense of purpose.

4. Provide Guidance and Mentorship:

- **Experienced Members:** Establish mentorship programs for experienced members to support those fresh to their wellness journey.
- **Knowledge Sharing:** Encourage the interchange of knowledge and expertise, fostering a culture of lifelong learning.

5. Celebrating Milestones:

- **Recognition:** Recognize and celebrate individual and communal accomplishments, such as meeting a fitness goal, conquering a challenge, or maintaining a healthy habit.
- **Collective Joy:** Share in the joy of others, fostering a sense of community and shared success.

The Effects of Supportive Communities on Wellbeing

1. Motivation and Inspiration:

- **Collective Energy:** A supportive community's combined energy can motivate individuals to push their limits and achieve personal best.
- **Inspiring experiences:** Hearing and experiencing the experiences of those who have overcome barriers or accomplished extraordinary feats can be a source of motivation.

2. Emotional Resilience:

- **Emotional Support:**A supportive group offers emotional support, empathy, and understanding during difficult times.
- **Shared Coping Mechanisms:** Members discuss coping methods and ideas for dealing with stress, which promotes emotional resilience.

3. Consistency and Accountability:

- **Consistency:** Community commitment to wellness goals fosters consistency by instilling a sense of responsibility for self and others.
- **Accountability Partnerships:** Forming accountability partnerships improves adherence to routines and goals.

4. Improving Mental Well-Being:

- **Reducing Isolation:** Belonging to a community lowers feelings of loneliness, which can negatively impact mental health.

- **Positive Affirmations:** Receiving regular positive affirmations and support from community members helps to foster a positive mindset.

5. Knowledge Exchange:

- **Holistic Learning:** Communities foster holistic learning by bringing together individuals with varied backgrounds to share views on nutrition, fitness, mental health, and well-being.
- **Preventing disinformation:** The exchange of factual information helps prevent the spread of disinformation, helping members to make educated choices.

Practical Strategies for Creating a Supportive Community

1. Establish clear guidelines:

- **Code of Conduct:** Create a clear code of conduct that values respect, inclusivity, and empathy.
- **Support criteria:** Establish clear criteria for offering constructive support and feedback.

2. Utilise Technology:

- **Online Platforms:** Leverage social media groups, forums, or dedicated apps to create virtual spaces where members can connect, share, and support each other.
- **Virtual Events:** Organize virtual events such as webinars, Q&A sessions, or group workouts to facilitate community engagement.

3. Foster Personal Connections:

- **Introductions and Icebreakers:** Organize introductions and icebreaker events to enable people to connect on a personal level.

- **Buddy Systems:** Set up buddy systems in which members are paired for mutual support and encouragement.

4. Regular Check-Ins and Updates:

- **Weekly updates:** Encourage participants to provide weekly updates on their progress, difficulties, and achievements.
- **Check-in Sessions:** Hold regular check-ins, either digitally or in person, to build a sense of community and mutual understanding.

5. Recognition Programs:

- **Member Spotlights:** Introduce member spotlights to showcase individual achievements and contributions to the community.
- **Recognition Awards:** Establish recognition awards for milestones, acts of support, or other notable contributions.

6. Wellness Challenges:

- **Collective Challenges:** Organize wellness challenges that members can participate in together, fostering a sense of collective achievement.
- **Prizes and Recognition:** Offer prizes or recognition for individuals and teams that excel in wellness challenges.

7. Professional Guidance:

- **Expert Involvement:** Bring in wellness experts, fitness trainers, or nutritionists to offer advice and answer questions from the community.
- **Workshops and Webinars:** Organise workshops and webinars on important wellness topics to expand the community's knowledge base.

Realizing the Vision: Success Stories from Supportive Communities

1. Transformational Narratives:

- **Weight loss journeys:** Share tales about community members who went on weight loss journeys, emphasizing the need for support in maintaining motivation.
- **Fitness Progressions:** Highlight individuals who made major fitness gains with the support of the community.

2. Overcoming Health issues:

- **Recovery experiences:** Share experiences of individuals who overcome health issues and highlight the importance of community support in their recovery.
- **Chronic Conditions:** Highlight members who are managing chronic conditions with the help of a caring and supportive community.

3. Mental Wellness Testimonials:

- **Stress Management:** Share how community members find successful stress management tactics with support and assistance.
- **Mental Health Advocacy:** Highlight those who advocate for mental health in the community, fostering a climate of free discussion.

4. Group Achievements:

- **Group Milestones:** Celebrate group accomplishments like running a distance, meeting fitness goals, or completing wellness challenges.
- **Community activities:** Highlight community-led activities, emphasizing the importance of collaborative efforts on individual and group success.

Evolving Your Meditation and Yoga Journey

In the tranquil landscapes of meditation and yoga, the trip is not a static destination, but rather a dynamic, ever-changing adventure of self-discovery and evolution. Beyond the serenity of silence and the fluidity of yoga poses is a profound journey—one that goes beyond physical movements and breath awareness, into the worlds of mental clarity, emotional resilience, and spiritual enlightenment.

Introduction to the Living Essence of Meditation and Yoga

Meditation and yoga are ancient pillars in the modern wellness tapestry, providing timeless insights and practices that have endured for generations. Despite their ancient origins, these practices are not trapped in time; rather, they are living traditions that adapt to and resonate with the ever-changing terrain of human experience. Evolving your meditation and yoga practice is not a break from tradition, but rather an intimate conversation with the essence of these practices—a conversation that encourages investigation, growth, and the uncovering of profound layers of self-awareness.

The Dynamics of Evolution: Adapting Your Practice.

1. Tailoring to Individual Needs

- **Body Awareness:** Tuning into your body's requirements is the first step towards evolving your practice. Recognize its signals, tailor postures to your specific anatomy, and welcome changes that promote your physical well-being.
- **Mindful Adjustments:** Listen to your body's responses when meditating. If a specific pose feels difficult or distracting, give yourself the freedom to change, ensuring that your practice remains a source of comfort and

peace.

2. Exploring Different Styles:

- **Variety in Yoga Practices:** Consider trying several types of yoga, from the dynamic flow of Vinyasa to the calm of Yin. Each style has a distinct flavor, allowing you to work different muscles, increase flexibility, and discover what resonates most deeply with your inner self.
- **Diversifying Meditation Techniques:** Meditation is not one-size-fits-all. Experiment with several meditation approaches, including mindfulness, loving-kindness, and transcendental meditation. This exploration assists you in determining the technique that best suits your temperament and goals.

3. Integrating Breathwork:

- **Conscious Breathing:** Developing your practice requires a stronger connection to breathwork. Investigate pranayama techniques in yoga, such as Ujjayi breath or Nadi Shodhana, to improve focus and energy levels. Use breath awareness to the ground and center yourself during meditation.
- **Breath as a Bridge:** Recognise the breath as a link between the physical and mental. Incorporate intention into your breathing, using it as a conduit for energy and awareness throughout your practice.

4. Mindful Transitions:

- **Seamless Integration:** Incorporate flowing transitions throughout your yoga practice instead of static poses. Embrace the gaps between positions, cultivating mindfulness in every step. This fluidity not only promotes physical flexibility but also facilitates a smooth transition to meditation.
- **Mindful Transitions in Meditation:** Apply mindfulness to the transitions between various meditation practices. Approach shifts from focused

attention to open awareness, or from seated meditation to walking meditation, with an intentional and mindful presence.

Deepening the Inner Landscape: Nurturing Meditation Journey

1. Learning Advanced Meditation Techniques:

- **Mantra Meditation:** Immerse yourself in mantra meditation, which focuses on the rhythmic chanting of sacred sounds or words. Mantra meditation improves attention, cultivates a sense of sacred resonance, and demonstrates the transformational power of sound vibrations.
- **Visualizations:** Include visualizations in your meditation practice. During meditation, visualize quiet landscapes, symbols of tranquility, or personal objectives to improve the imaginative and creative aspects of your practice.

2. Practice Silence and Stillness:

- **Extend quiet Meditation:** Gradually increase the duration of quiet meditation. Embracing lengthier periods of quiet allows for a deeper inner journey, revealing layers of mental chatter and cultivating a calm frame of mind.
- **Stillness in Yoga Positions:** Holding postures for longer periods will help you deepen your yoga practice. The quietness encourages a meditative character, increasing awareness of physiological sensations and allowing for a meditative flow between positions.

3. Integrating Mindfulness into Daily Life:

- **Mindful Daily Activities:** Increase the depth of your meditation by incorporating awareness into daily tasks. Whether it's mindful dining, strolling, or even dishwashing, infuse these experiences with present-moment awareness to go beyond the typical bounds of formal meditation.
- **Moment-to-Moment Awareness:** In yoga, graduate from asana practice

to embody mindfulness in everyday movements. Incorporate the principles of alignment, breath awareness, and presence into everyday tasks to cultivate a consistent thread of mindfulness throughout the day.

4. Exploring Meditation Retreats :

- **Immersive Experiences:** Consider attending meditation retreats to gain immersive experiences. These retreats offer a favorable atmosphere for deepening your practice, direction from experienced instructors, and the formation of a supportive community of fellow practitioners.
- **Integration in Daily Life:** After returning from a retreat, use the insights acquired into your daily life. Whether it's sticking to a steady meditation schedule, implementing mindfulness practices, or developing a feeling of community, the retreat experience catalyzes long-term growth.

Synchronizing Meditation and Yoga: Creating Harmony

1. Unified Breath and Movement:

- **Breath-Centric Asana Practice:** Evolve your yoga practice by focusing on the breath. Allow the breath to lead your motions, resulting in a fluid dance of breath and posture. This synchronization enhances the contemplative nature of the practice.
- **Mindful transitions in yoga:** Incorporate a sense of mindfulness into each transition as you move through the yoga sequences. Recognize the interplay of breath, movement, and consciousness, resulting in a harmonic symphony that transcends physical poses.

2. Chakra Meditation in Yoga:

- **Chakra Alignment:** Incorporate chakra meditation into your yoga practice. As you progress through the postures, imagine the alignment and activation of the energy centers along the spine. This holistic method balances the physical and energetic aspects of your practice.

- **Energetic Flow in Yoga:** Allow chakra awareness to guide the flow of energy in yoga. Visualize the upward passage of energy during inhale and its grounding descent during exhale to build a deep connection between body, mind, and soul.

3. Using Mudras:

- **Mudras for Meditation:** Mudras, or symbolic hand motions that alter energy flow, can help you deepen your meditation. Each mudra has a distinct meaning and effect, such as increasing attention and channeling spiritual energy.
- **Mudras for Yoga:** Include mudras in your yoga practice, particularly during seated postures and meditation-in-motion sequences. The intentional use of mudras adds a symbolic and contemplative component to the physical exercise.

4. Yoga Nidra for Deep Relaxation:

- **Guided Relaxation:** Integrate Yoga Nidra, or guided relaxation, into your meditation practice. This approach causes conscious relaxation, which allows for a profound release of bodily and mental tension.
- **Transcending Stress in Yoga:** Incorporate conscious relaxation between postures or at the end of your practice. Accept the meditative aspect of stillness, enabling the body to reap the benefits of the practice.

Cultivating Evolution of Mind, Body, and Spirit

1. Mindful Nutrition:

- **Conscious eating:** Increase your well-being by incorporating mindfulness into your eating habits. Practice mindful eating, savoring each bite, and feeling grateful for the nourishment supplied. This mindfulness enhances the meditative and mindful components of your yoga and meditation activities.

2. Journaling for Reflection:

- **Reflective Practice:** Develop self-awareness through journaling. After your meditation or yoga sessions, spend some time reflecting on your experiences, insights, and feelings. This reflective practice becomes an important tool for tracking your progress and getting insight about your trip.

3. Connecting with Community:

- **Satsang and Sangha:** Connect with like-minded people through Satsang (spiritual conversation) or sangha (community). Connecting with a supportive group, whether in person or virtually, brings inspiration, shared ideas, and a sense of belonging, all of which promote the progression of your practice.

4. Spiritual Exploration:

- **Study Sacred Texts:** Learn about the knowledge of yoga and meditation. Studying writings such as the Bhagavad Gita, Yoga Sutras, or mindfulness literature broadens your understanding and offers guidance for a more in-depth examination of your spiritual path.
- **getting Guidance:** Consider getting advice from spiritual mentors, teachers, or advanced practitioners. Their ideas and experiences might provide valuable perspectives, sparking fresh directions in your path.

10

CONCLUSION

Encouragement for the Continued Path Ahead

In the broad tapestry of life, the trip ahead is a never-ending path that winds through peaks of delight, and valleys of adversity, and provides a landscape for self-discovery. As we stand at the crossroads of the present moment, the encouragement to continue on the path ahead serves as a beacon, illuminating the way forward.

The Eternal Dance of Progress.

The road ahead is a dynamic dance—a rhythmic interplay of progress, setbacks, and the ability to accept both. Encouragement for the trip ahead is more than just a motivational boost; it is a recognition of the underlying strength inside, a reminder that the seeds of potential await to grow with each step taken.

1. Embracing the Journey:

- **Not Just the Destination:** Living in the Present: The motivation to persevere stems from a deep realization that the journey itself is the destination. Embrace the present moment, savoring its richness and realizing that each step adds to your life's evolving tale.

- **Learning from diversions:** Understand that diversions and unexpected turns are necessary for the path. Instead of seeing them as hurdles, consider them chances for growth and learning that will add depth to your life's tapestry.

2. Resilience in the Face of Challenges:

- **Viewing challenges as catalysts:** Challenges are not impediments to growth; rather, they serve as catalysts. The encouragement comes from viewing setbacks as stepping stones, moving you ahead with fresh power and perseverance.
- **Celebrating Small Wins:** Small achievements should be celebrated even in the face of adversity. Every accomplishment, no matter how small, demonstrates your ability to conquer challenges. These wins serve as the foundation for long-term encouragement.

3. The Importance of Self-Compassion:

- **Accepting Imperfection:** Self-compassion inspires hope for the future. Accept your flaws and vulnerabilities, knowing that they are woven into the fabric of your individual experience.
- **Affirming self-worth:** Affirm your self-worth regardless of external affirmation. The trip ahead gets easier when you grasp that your innate value transcends achievements and external expectations.

4. Developing Internal Strength:

- **Cultivating Intrinsic Motivation:** Intrinsic motivation drives persistence. Connect with the interests and ideals that drive your journey, and tap into the source of power that comes from pursuing what is truly important to you.

- **Recognizing Inner Resilience:** Consider previous occasions where inner resilience prevailed. Whether you're fighting adversity, chasing aspirations, or adapting to change, remember the inner strength that has carried you through.

5. Developing a Growth Mindset:

- **Embracing Change for Growth:** Encouragement flourishes in a developing attitude. Change should be viewed as an opportunity for learning and progress, rather than a threat. Accept obstacles with a desire to learn, cultivating a mindset that sees failures as opportunities for growth.
- **Learning From Setbacks:** Instead of perceiving setbacks as failures, see them as great lessons. Each diversion or challenge allows for introspection, learning, and adaptation, which is an important part of the trip ahead.

6. Navigating Uncertainty with Courage:

- **Courage to Embrace Uncertainty:** The encouragement comes from having the bravery to journey into the unknown, believing that each stride forward, even in the face of uncertainty, is a step towards self-discovery and growth.
- **Developing a Supportive Mindset:** Develop a mindset that sees uncertainty as an opportunity rather than a threat. Consider the journey ahead as an adventure full of surprises and chances waiting to be discovered.

7. Building a Supportive Network:

- **Surrounding Yourself with Positivity:** Encouragement is amplified in the presence of supporting people. Create a network of good influences—friends, family, and mentors—who will encourage and motivate you on your quest.
- **Sharing Aspirations:** Openly discuss your goals and challenges with your

support group. Sharing develops a sense of accountability, friendship, and mutual encouragement as you journey forward together.

8. Reconnecting with Passion and Purpose:

- **Rediscovering Passion:** Rediscovering your passions can inspire you to keep going. Consider the hobbies, pursuits, or causes that kindle a spark within you, imbuing your journey with meaning and energy.
- **Aligning with core values:** Connect to your essential principles. Ensure that the path ahead is consistent with these beliefs, establishing a roadmap that reflects your true self and creates a feeling of purposeful direction.

9. Celebrating the Journey's Diversity:

- **Valuing Diverse Experiences:** Encouragement develops as we embrace the variety of experiences that the journey provides. Each phase, whether smooth or difficult, adds to the depth of your story. Celebrate the variety of events as important chapters in your particular journey.
- **Finding delight in the Process:** Instead of fixating on distant goals, find delight in the process. The motivation to keep going is increased when each step becomes an opportunity to enjoy the current moment, finding fulfillment in the journey itself.

10. Cultivating Mindfulness and Reflection:

- **Mindful Presence:** Encouragement comes from aware presence. Cultivate a mindfulness practice by savoring the beauty of each moment and allowing the journey ahead to unfold with awareness.
- **Reflecting on Growth:** Regularly reflecting on your progress can be a tremendous source of motivation. Recognize your progress, perseverance, and lessons learned; reflection brings clarity, supporting your ability to navigate the route ahead.